Hypnosis for Smoking Cessation

An NLP and Hypnotherapy Practitioner's Manual

David Botsford

Crown House Publishing Limited

www.crownhouse.co.uk
www.chpus.com

First published by

Crown House Publishing Ltd
Crown Buildings, Bancyfelin, Carmarthen, Wales, SA33 5ND, UK
www.crownhouse.co.uk

and

Crown House Publishing Company LLC
6 Trowbridge Drive, Suite 5, Bethel, CT 06801-2858, USA
www.CHPUS.com

British Library Cataloguing-in-Publication Data
A catalogue entry for this book is available
from the British Library.

ISBN 978-184590074-8

LCCN 2007925539

Printed and bound in the USA

To my clients, for what they have taught me.

Contents

Accompanying CD-ROM
1   Client Handout, short form
2   Client Handout, long form
3   Transcripts from two actual sessions

Acknowledgements

Many people have made this volume possible. Particular thanks are due to all the hypnotherapists who have attended the seminars on smoking cessation which produced the raw material from which the book was written. I would like to thank Patrick Doherty, Ed McArthur and Hugh Marley for their invaluable help with the seminars, Wendy Pilkington for transcribing the therapy sessions which are included on the CD-Rom, and Ron Alexander for his idea of putting the material together in the form of a book and encouragement for the writing of it. Thanks also to Roy Hunter for his useful comments on an early version of the manuscript, which have been incorporated in the final version. The vision, expertise and support of everybody at Crown House Publishing has also been priceless, and is greatly appreciated.

The hypnotherapist and the smoking habit

Let me begin by making a point of central importance. The client who visits a hypnotherapist to stop smoking is not coming to be hypnotised. The client is coming in order to become a non-smoker. The hypnotherapist's goal is to communicate in whatever way it takes to ensure that the client both becomes a non-smoker and knows how to stay one permanently. When someone becomes a non-smoker, there is always some kind of breakthrough, a moment of transformation, an epiphany, in which the change happens. Before this moment, that person was a smoker; afterwards, they are a non-smoker. This moment might come before, during or after the time when the client is in hypnotic trance.

Heed the point being made here. Hypnotic trance is an extraordinarily powerful means of bringing about the transformation which enables a person to stop smoking. Yet the hypnotherapist must actively work to optimise all the elements which influence the client, not knowing exactly when that breakthrough will take place.

In order to illustrate this point, let us turn to the frank and entertaining memoirs of the late Allen Carr. Mr Carr was a chartered accountant who smoked no fewer than 100 cigarettes a day. Having gained a powerful insight which enabled him to become a non-smoker, he wrote the best-selling book *The Easy Way to Stop Smoking* and ran seminars which have enabled millions around the world to successfully quit smoking. He became the best-known smoking cessation expert in the United Kingdom, if not the world.

In his autobiography, he describes how his father, a heavy smoker, was dying of lung cancer in hospital at the age of 56:

> "His last words to me were to make me promise to quit smoking. I made that promise without hesitation. I'd already decided that no way would I end up like him. The moment I left the hospital, I lit a cigarette."[1]

Here is the first essential point to take on board. Negative experiences are usually counterproductive in achieving smoking cessation. Even when a person does stop smoking as a result of an experience such as a close relative dying of a smoking-related illness, it generally lasts only a short time. Negative experiences tend to set off chain reactions in which people become disempowered and unresourceful, and often engage in self-destructive behaviour. Time and again, clients of mine have described how they had successfully quit smoking for several years. Then they get divorced, lose their job, learn that a relative is severely ill or find their business is going bankrupt, and immediately they light a cigarette. As the body tastes that cigarette, it recalls the many years of smoking during which they may have consumed ten, twenty or thirty cigarettes a day. The body assumes that the person is going back to the smoking habit, and reverts to the earlier smoking pattern, once again demanding ten, twenty or thirty cigarettes a day.

Effective hypnotherapy for smoking cessation depends entirely on the use of positive messages and experiences. The goal is to empower clients, so that they may draw on their own resourcefulness, and use their knowledge for personal transformation, thus setting up a positive chain reaction. Now they can focus on the benefits of being a non-smoker, and experience themselves as capable, resourceful individuals who are now achieving success in quitting smoking. The hypnotherapist should look on the consulting room as a "sacred space" where no negative influences are allowed to linger. The hypnotherapist must communicate in positive terms, and "reframe" any negative talk from the client in equally positive terms.

Carr describes how he later became so ill from smoking that he was coughing up blood, yet still could not quit the habit. His wife Joyce urged him to visit a hypnotherapist. Carr recalls:

> "I was very dubious. … I was certain hypnotherapy was not the answer and that the whole exercise would be a waste of time and money. No one could kid me that I didn't need to smoke. But I agreed to go, purely to placate Joyce. I wanted to be able to say to her: 'Look, I've done what you asked, but it hasn't worked!'

> "I didn't set out with the deliberate intention of resisting the hypnotherapist's influence. If he could have cured me, I would have been prepared to pretend I was a chicken or suffer any indignity he might suggest. I knew smoking was going to kill me and expected it to happen soon. This knowledge made me want to quit, but it didn't enable me to do it, any more than watching my father die of lung cancer had made me break nicotine's spell either …

> "That day started with me a picture of abject misery. Who could have predicted that it would end up the greatest day of my life?"[2]

Carr's beliefs and future-pacing before the session were far from ideal for achieving a successful result. In NLP, *future-pacing* is defined as "the process of mentally rehearsing some future situation in order to help ensure that the desired behaviour will occur naturally and automatically." Note that the intellectual knowledge of the dangers of smoking caused Carr to consciously want to stop smoking, but this had no effect on his behaviour, because behaviour is governed by the unconscious mind.

Carr describes his visit to the hypnotherapist:

"I had anticipated being met by an individual straight out of a Hollywood film, with bushy eyebrows, piercing eyes and a goatee beard. To my relief, what I got was a bright, earnest, clean-shaven young man. Before the therapy we had a friendly chat about smoking generally, during the course of which the smidgen was added:

"'Do you realize that smoking is just nicotine addiction and if you quit for long enough you will eventually be free?'

"I cannot remember another statement he made during our chat, but that smidgen – that smoking is just nicotine addiction – remained lodged in my brain. … Now, seeing myself in this new light, as someone addicted to a drug, I believed the goal of quitting was achievable."[3]

This insight led Carr to realise that all that smoking a cigarette does for the smoker is relieve the effect of the nicotine from the previous cigarette. The cigarette provides no pleasure or enjoyment. If the smoker recognises that fact and allows the nicotine to pass out of the body, the cycle is broken and the smoker quits the habit. This flash of inspiration became the basis of his Easyway smoking cessation system which has freed millions from the tobacco habit.

Carr continues his recollection of that session:

"It seemed a bit late to be springing news of my conversion on the hypnotherapist, and so I kept quiet. The session was now pointless, but as long as he didn't become aware of this fact there would be little harm in going through with it. I was asked to close my eyes and imagine I was walking through a beautiful garden. This I did and very pleasant it was too. Then I was told my left arm would begin to feel very light, it would become lighter and lighter and eventually weightless and float in mid air. Ten minutes of cajoling didn't make it feel any lighter and my growing embarrassment for the therapist blocked out all possibility of relaxation. I seriously considered cheating just to get a result but decided against it.

"Eventually he gave up and asked me to open my eyes. He decided on another tack, explaining that certain techniques worked better with some people than with others. This time he held a pencil about a foot from my nose and in a monotonous chant told me how my eyelids would gradually become heavier and heavier until I could no longer keep my eyes open. I'd never felt more awake in my life. Seeing the consternation on the young man's face as this technique went the way of the first was excruciating. I decided to bring the farce to an end as quickly as possible, and closed my eyes. It took a further fifteen minutes for him to deliver a string of platitudes about the futility of smoking. All I could think about was escaping outside for a smoke.

"I lit up the moment I left the clinic and make my way home, that statement – my catalyst for quitting – still going round inside my head."[4]

Carr returned home and read a medical textbook which explained the effects of smoking on the body, in the light of the insight he had gained during the session. He recalled:

"The startling fact I discovered was that when nicotine leaves your body it creates an empty, insecure feeling. By smoking another cigarette you replace the nicotine and get rid of that feeling, which leaves you feeling less nervous or more relaxed than you did the moment before you lit up. ... The catalyst and seed of what would become Easyway had fused in my brain."[5]

It is worth examining this account for the lessons it provides. Quite possibly, it was the most successful smoking cessation hypnotherapy session of all time.

From the point of view of hypnotherapeutic technique, it left considerable scope for improvement. As a means of inducing trance, the hypnotherapist asks Carr to imagine walking through a garden. A more effective way to induce trance is to ask the client to describe a memory of a situation in which he felt relaxed, and then feed back and elaborate on the client's description. An actual memory is far more real than an imaginary situation. The client, not the therapist, should select the relaxed situation. Not every client necessarily likes or can connect with the concept of being in a garden.

Then the therapist attempts to gain unconscious arm levitation, an ideomotor response, by making suggestions for no less than *ten minutes*! First, it is important to follow "the three second rule": if a client is not responding to a technique or suggestion after three seconds, simply say, "That's fine," and move on to a different approach. Any attempt to keep a technique going for longer when the client is not responding is likely to destroy the credibility of the entire session. Second, attempting to achieve hypnotic phenomena such as an ideomotor response or eye catalepsy is pointless. The client is not paying good money to have their arms going up and down like a windmill, or to be unable to open their eyes. If these phenomena are achieved, they do nothing to enable the client to stop smoking. If they are not achieved, then the client is likely to assume that the whole session is useless and that hypnotherapy is ineffective. Either way, valuable time which can be put to far better use has been taken up. Omit such things completely. The client is paying to become a non-smoker, so make sure that every minute of the session is devoted to achieving that goal.

Then the therapist attempts to induce trance by displaying a pencil as an object of fixation and making suggestions for eye closure. An object of fixation which the client internally visualises is more effective in trance induction than an external, physical one. Milton H. Erickson, the psychiatrist who was history's greatest medical hypnotherapist, carried out scientific experiments with real and imagined crystal balls, metronomes, pendulums and other apparatus used as objects of fixation. He found that:

> "Numerous experiments … in which … subjects watched silent pendulums or listened to soft music or to metronomes disclosed that imaginary aids were much more effective than actual apparatus. … The utilization of imagery rather than actual apparatus permits the subjects to utilize their actual capabilities without being hampered by an adjustment to nonessential externalities."[6]

Erickson summarises his subjects' comments as follows:

> "When I listen to the imaginary metronome, it speeds up or slows down, gets louder or fainter, as I start to go into a trance, and I just drift along. With the real metronome, it remains distractingly constant, and it keeps pulling me back to reality instead of letting me drift along into a trance. The imaginary metronome is changeable and always fits in with just the way I'm thinking and feeling, but I have to fit myself to the real one."[7]

When using an object of fixation, use an imagined one rather than a physical one. (This does not contradict what was said above about memories, where real memories are more effective than imagined situations.)

Then the therapist makes suggestions for eye closure and Carr recalls that "I'd never felt more awake in my life." First, eye closure is advantageous but not essential for trance. It cuts off the external visual field, and therefore reduces the risk of distraction. The hypnotherapist does better to say something like, "And those eyes can close any time they want," or "And can you experience that more easily with your eyes opened or *closed*?", with a slight emphasis on the last word. That way, whether the eyes close or stay open, rapport is maintained and the client's response is consistent with the therapist's words. If the client's eyes close, all to the good; if not, simply proceed with them open.

Then the therapist gave "platitudes about the futility of smoking." In trance, it is vital to talk about the constructive things you *do* want the client to achieve, rather than what you want them to avoid. The client already knows, intellectually, that smoking is futile; the therapist needs to achieve the positive goal the client does want, and create a context in which the client's unconscious finds the solution which makes that goal a reality.

Yet the therapist must be congratulated on the result he achieved right at the start, even before the therapy officially began. Hypnosis has been defined as "the subconscious realisation of an idea". During the initial friendly chat "before" the therapy, the hypnotherapist conveyed, in ordinary conversation, with the client in full waking awareness, an idea of immense power. That idea became a catalyst which mobilised Carr's creative faculty and enabled him to understand the reality of smoking and how to break free from it. He went on to communicate that idea to millions and help them, too, become non-smokers.

The client is a unique, resourceful individual, capable of learning in many different ways. The hypnotherapist's task is to educate clients, to mobilise their creative faculties for finding the way to quit smoking, and to train them in techniques which enable them to stay non-smokers in all situations. Inducing trance and making suggestions to stop smoking are important, but making suggestions is only one factor among several that are equally vital. As Erickson explained:

> "Your purpose in using hypnosis is to communicate ideas and understandings and to get the patient to utilize the competencies that exist within him at both a psychological level and a physiological level."[8]

Every client has a vast treasure trove of competencies or resources, which they have been acquiring throughout their life. The hypnotherapist's task is to remind the client of this wealth of expertise and to lead the client to a context in which they can creatively apply those resources to the task of becoming a non-smoker.

Chapter 1

The elements of transformation

A story about smoking cessation

When he was eight years old, Stuart's class at school had a film show. It was a 16mm projector in those days, and the children were most impressed that the film was in colour. Stuart was absorbed by a fascinating story about a group of children just like him, who lived in a town just like his, encountering the smoking menace. Later, he struggled to recall the details of the plot. He did remember a sinister but plausible villain who attempted to coax the kids into smoking cigarettes. The one scene that did stick in his mind, even decades later, was when the children secretly followed the villain to his lair – a rubble-strewn building site behind a brick wall. Behind the wall was a monstrous contraption worthy of W. Heath Robinson himself. At one end a lighted cigarette was being smoked by what looked like a huge set of bellows, perpetually opening and closing, drawing the smoke in and through a complex array of glass tubes down into several transparent flasks, the sort used in chemistry experiments. One flask contained a thick mud of black tar, another a heap of ash, a third was stained by brown nicotine and a fourth was green with radioactive materials. The children in the film – and those in the classroom – looked in awestruck horror at this formidable collection of poisons accumulated at the bottom of the machine. All determined that they would stay non-smokers for life.

For about six years after that, thoughts about cigarettes hardly intruded at all on Stuart's mind. But soon after he started at secondary school, a few of his friends – including those who had seen that same anti-smoking film – started smoking their first cigarettes. By the age of 13, several of them were confirmed smokers. Stuart actually held out against the habit longer than most. At school, tempted by his friends, he tried smoking one cigarette but found it so revolting it put him off. But the idea had been planted.

It was during the long summer holidays, when he was 14, that Stuart became a smoker. He was staying with his slightly older cousins, whom he had always looked up to, at their farmhouse. During those warm, idyllic evenings, well out of view of both sets of parents, Stuart had ample leisure time for overcoming the coughing, the dizziness, the nausea and the burning sensation in his mouth and lungs. Day after day, inhaling deeper and deeper, Stuart's body gradually adapted to the new habit. By the time he returned to school in September, Stuart didn't need to think about it any more – he was already on ten a day. His smoking friends at school were most impressed by his achievement. Somehow he managed to keep the secret from his parents for almost a whole year.

Content with the habit, he left school and went to college, where the smoking habit proved most useful. It was a ticket to membership of the gregarious, trendy set who stayed up till five in the morning. Often he would smoke twenty, thirty, even forty cigarettes over twenty-four hours. He remained in excellent health, and even took part in college sports.

Once he left college and started his career, the smoking habit still proved to be an asset. His immediate manager smoked, several of his closest colleagues smoked, and most importantly, the big boss smoked. Every break, they could be found in a little circle outside the front entrance. The loud laughter from the exchange of news and gossip evoked curiosity and even a twinge of envy from the non-smokers inside, isolated from the grapevine.

The propaganda against smoking was distant thunder. His health remained excellent. Now and then he faced funny looks when smoking in certain places, but otherwise he was satisfied with his habit.

Things only started to change after his thirtieth birthday. His fiancée, who had already quit smoking, vaguely hinted that she wanted him to give up as well. His new employer frowned on the habit, and at the new firm he found himself outside with a very different group than before. Now and again he got the distinct impression that he was getting out of breath much more quickly than he should have been. Several of his best friends were trying to quit, some more successfully than others. What surprised him most was that when he went to visit his cousins out in the country, they had actually quit smoking and he even had to ask them to hunt for an ashtray when he lit up.

So the idea of becoming a non-smoker became a firmer intention. He set the date and stopped through sheer willpower. But the cravings made him irritable, and the thought of cigarettes was on his mind day and night. Reverting to smoking was the path of least resistance, and he took that path. He was determined to try again some time – perhaps in the New Year. As soon as the pharmacist opened on 2nd January, he went in and bought some nicotine patches. For several weeks of wearing the patches, he did stop, and got to the point where he removed the final patch. For a month or so, he was a non-smoker, and welcomed the change.

But it wasn't to last. This was a time of economic downturn, and people at work were being given the sack. Stuart was one of the luckier ones, but he found his workload massively increased as he took on the work of those who had lost their jobs. His stress levels increased dramatically, and he found himself cadging a cigarette from one of the firm's die-hard smokers. After that, it was only a few days before he was back on twenty a day. Even though his employers sent him on a stress management course, where he learned how to get his stress levels under control, he continued smoking.

As the firm's prospects picked up again, and new recruits took on some of the workload, Stuart began thinking about quitting again. He was about to get married and had to start thinking seriously about his long-term health. After the wedding, when they moved into the new house, *then* he would quit.

So he did. There was a single moment when it all came together. Just sitting there in the garden of an evening, thinking about all the months they had worked to prepare the house, Stuart experienced a remarkable sense of ease and comfort. He lost track of time, experiencing "eternity in a moment", while his mind wandered freely through his memories and imagination. Once again he vividly saw that monstrous contraption from that childhood film show. He saw himself – as an adult – removing the lit cigarette from that machine and stubbing it out against the brick wall. He imagined himself emptying those transparent flasks of the tar, nicotine, ash and radioactive materials, and washing them clean. Then he watched that contraption "breathing" clean and fresh air, and he sensed an extraordinary feeling of freedom, ease and connection with life coming from some inner intelligence.

After that, he simply forgot about that old habit. He lived life much the way he had before, and felt as if a massive shift of energy had taken place within. After two weeks, when the accumulated poison had left his body, he found that his stamina improved and his senses sharpened. Cigarette smoke now irritated his eyes, smelt horrible and made him want to cough. As the film of tar disappeared from the top of his tongue, food tasted better. And by committing to regular exercise, he was able to remain slim. He could handle difficult work situations, socialise, relax in the evenings, enjoy a meal and even have a drink with smokers, and enjoy all these situations with his new sense of independence.

Asked how he would describe this transformation, he replied that he felt a greater awareness of his body and its sensations, a greater sense of his own worth, a more harmonious connection with other people, and a greater sense of optimism about the future. He compared it to many things he had learned to do in the past: mastering sports, gaining skills and increased pay at his job, learning to drive. This new experience of healthy living simply became a permanent part of who he now was.

Learning to be a non-smoker

The above story is a composite based on the experiences of numerous hypnotherapy clients. The one part that comes from my own experience is the description of the anti-smoking film and its impact on me. It inoculated me against smoking so much that I have never smoked more than one drag on a cigarette, and even then only as a teenager under severe pressure from peers.

My original interest in hypnotherapy was its role as a rapid form of therapy – enabling an individual to transform their life in just a few sessions, and mind-body healing – accessing unconscious resources to achieve physical well-being. However, when I set up as a hypnotherapist, the largest group who wanted to avail themselves of my services were people who wanted to quit smoking. At an early stage in my career as a hypnotherapist, I realised that if I were to achieve that particular goal, I would have to do two things. First, I would have to do whatever it took to enable the client to quit smoking in the session, using hypnotic trance to communicate with the client's unconscious mind. Second, I would need to teach the client to remain a non-smoker in every possible situation by gaining control over their subjective experience in the moment. This book describes exactly the methods I use to do both those tasks.

Chapter 2

The nature and function of trance

Trance is central to the way human beings make sense of and function in the world. At any given moment, our conscious attention is focused on certain objects while others are outside of awareness.

As we go through the day, we experience what are known as ultradian rhythms, in which the body and mind go through changes in psychological, physical, motor, perceptual and more complex social behaviour. Ultradian cycles are recurrent rhythms of less than twenty-four hours. Many ultradian rhythms are synchronised on a single ninety-minute cycle known as the basic rest activity cycle (BRAC). We spend ninety minutes focused on external realities, and then our awareness spontaneously "goes inside".

The psychologist Ernest Rossi observed that Milton Erickson utilised these naturally-occurring moments during ultradian rhythms as the optimum time to induce hypnosis for therapeutic change. Rossi noted that Erickson

> "would usually wait for the patient's physical and mental processes to 'quiet down' before he induced trance, explaining that he was waiting to utilize those 'natural' periods of quietness and receptivity. We soon began to call these quiet periods the 'common everyday trance' … because it seemed they were part of natural everyday life. The housewife staring vacantly over a cup of coffee, the student with a faraway look in his eyes during the middle of a lecture, and the driver who automatically reaches his destination with no memory of the details of his route, are all varieties of the common everyday trance."[1]

Trance can be experienced when absorbed in a hobby, reading a book or watching a film or play. Everything except the object of attention is excluded from awareness. In trance, the critical or analytical conscious mind is bypassed and spontaneous behaviours take place which would normally be inhibited by the conscious mind. For example, Shakespeare's *Othello* has a long history of audience intervention. In the scene where Iago seeks to convince Othello that Desdemona has been unfaithful – putting him in a trance, in fact – members of the audience have often shouted out to Othello that Iago is trying to deceive him.

People entering supermarkets enter a "shopper's trance". At the Market Research Society's conference in Brighton in 1988, two investigators described how they had studied this phenomenon. They hypnotised shoppers and found that they had a much better recall of the supermarket's brand information than they had when questioned in full waking awareness – which helps to show why some people's preferences, recorded in the standard clipboard interview, are often misleading.[2] If you have ever left a retail store having bought a lot more than you intended when you went in, you will know the power of "shopper's trance". Your purchases were made largely outside of conscious awareness.

Trance can be understood as the selective awareness of reality. Some people believe that everything in human experience is trance, while others argue that there is no such thing as trance. Ultimately, this debate cannot be resolved, because the word "trance" is merely a label that might – or might not – be placed on certain aspects of our experience.

The human senses take in only a small proportion of the vast amount of data present in the electro-magnetic spectrum. For example, most insects can see ultraviolet – which is how they find flowers. We need electronic devices to convert infra-red and ultra-violet light into forms that we can see. Even the data that our senses do detect goes through internal "filters" which classify it in terms of what we already know before consciousness integrates it into our model of the world. Without our ability to focus on selected parts of external reality, we would be overwhelmed by the flood of sensory data.

As we go through life, we develop habits and learnings which move from conscious to unconscious knowledge. A child learning to put shoes on and remove them goes through a process of conscious learning, in which the child has to learn to sit in a particular position, coordinate the shoe and the foot in putting them on, ensure that the tongue is in the correct position, tie shoelaces, and then untie the knots and remove the shoes. The child also learns to adapt to the tension and pressure of the shoes on their feet. After repeating these actions enough times, the child does them automatically, and the conscious mind ceases to notice the feel of the shoes on the feet. The unconscious mind has taken over the process of putting on, wearing and removing shoes. Because the unconscious mind has taken over these shoe-related tasks, the individual never needs to relearn them. The conscious mind is free to focus on new tasks. If unconscious actions are considered to be a phenomenon of trance, then one could say that the child has entered a "correct shoe-wearing" trance.

Indeed, in order to make sense of the above paragraph, you had to go into a "reading trance". When you first learned to read, you learned the letters of the alphabet, and then words, in conscious learning. Then the learning became unconscious. In reading the above passage, you may have experienced a positive hallucination of a young child learning to cope with shoes, and perhaps pseudo-orientation in time as you remember learning to use some hitherto unfamiliar item. Your conscious mind did not need to think about the letters of the alphabet or the words on this page at all.

Not all such "trances" are as useful as those which enable the mastery of shoes or reading. People can often put themselves into a trance which leads them into an unresourceful state. Consider someone who is expecting their partner home, but the partner is late. They start worrying, and this leads to a train of thought in which they imagine an accident, and a traumatic visit to the hospital – and then perhaps a funeral and how they are going to survive on their own. The psychotherapist Stephen Wolinsky describes how a person experiencing such anxiety is in an "anxiety trance":

> "Anxiety is a fear of the future. A client whose presenting problem is anxiety might be using a cluster of Deep Trance Phenomena to synthesize the sensation of anxiety. First comes *pseudo-orientation in time* as she imagines a catastrophic outcome occurring in the future and therefore experiences fear. Next she uses *posthypnotic suggestions* ("It will never work out," "I can't cope with life," "Nothing will help") to articulate and differentiate the particulars of the negative outcome she is imagining. These are reinforced by *negative hallucinations*, which block her ability to see or acknowledge other resources, and perhaps vivified by *positive hallucinations* as she visualizes herself encountering an anxiety-provoking stimulus (such as a bill collector) that is not present in present time. All of this turmoil is likely to be further exacerbated by an experience of *time distortion* in which she has a breathless feeling that there is not enough time to find any kind of solution."[3]

Becoming a smoker is also a way of achieving unconscious learning. For most people, it is a real ordeal to smoke their first few cigarettes. They taste and smell horrible. The smoke irritates the eyes. The body resists the incoming smoke by coughing, nausea, light-headedness and possibly vomiting. The presence of nicotine also causes a release of endorphins and endomorphines – the body's natural pain relievers – in order to ease the pain caused in resisting the poison from the cigarette. For most smokers, it takes real effort and commitment to persevere through this experience. Eventually, however, the body comes to expect the regular intake of cigarette smoke, the habit becomes unconscious, and the person has entered the "smoking trance".

People usually start smoking in order to achieve a resolution to some problem – about who they are, how they fit into society, and how they can become a member of a group. These problems confront every human being, and given the variability of human beings, they will create innumerable ways to solve them. One of these ways – which looked at in hindsight seems to be a kind of "quick fix" – is to start smoking.

Every problem was once a solution

Because the world is so complex, a habit we adopt as a solution in one context can become a problem to be solved in a different context. Smoking is deemed a solution because its associational or symbolic significance makes sense at the level of mind and meaning. The cigarette becomes a emblem or symbol of positive benefits, such as membership of a social group, of being grown-up, of proving oneself, of rebelling against authority, or of being cool, glamorous and sophisticated. This *positive hallucination* is as ridiculous as anything achieved in a stage hypnosis show. Yet the person takes up smoking in the belief that it will achieve those things. In doing so, they engage in the *negative hallucination* of blocking out anti-smoking health education messages and all knowledge about people who have suffered ill-health or early death from smoking. The body initially responds to the damage caused by the smoke with coughing, dizziness, nausea, watering eyes and perhaps vomiting. The novice smoker overrides these defensive reactions by smoking so many cigarettes that the body habituates to smoking and experiences it as normal. That is an example of *hypnotic anaesthesia*. As the smoking habit becomes unconscious, some smokers have a lit cigarette in the mouth first thing in the morning before they even open their eyes. That is an *ideomotor response*. The smoker's mind, too, is captured by the habit: the flow of thoughts is dominated by words, images and feelings connected with the smoking habit. These include *autosuggestions* ("Lunchtime – time for a cigarette"), *post-hypnotic suggestions* ("I'll buy a pack of twenty from that shop on the way home"), and *future-pacing* ("It'll be miserable not being able to smoke on that flight to Australia").

The hypnotherapist's task is to empower the client to break out of the "smoking trance" and to move them forward to a new representation of themselves and their relationship with the world, in which they find new and more useful ways to achieve the purposes of the unconscious than through the smoking habit. This new identity is not quite the same as their experience in the years before smoking the first cigarette. Even after having successfully quit smoking, the representation of the smoking habit is still there in the unconscious, but it has a different meaning. However, it is as irrelevant to the person's current life as many other interests they have left in the past.

Should an ex-smoker smoke just one cigarette, they will quickly re-enter the "smoking trance" as the body reverts to its memory of the years of smoking. Therefore, as well as enabling the client to quit smoking during the session, it is essential to teach the client how to stay free from the risk of reverting to the "smoking trance".

The client's power of creativity enables them to shift from one trance to another. Creativity is about forming new connections between two or more hitherto unconnected ideas or concepts. The client already has the resources which will enable them to become a non-smoker. The hypnotherapist's task then is to lead the client to the creative state which will enable them to make new associations in their own unique way. What is usually described as "hypnotic trance" is more of a creative experience which acts as a bridge between the trance which the client has experienced up till now, and which is now recognised to be disempowering, and the more useful trance which they will experience in the future. Smoking cessation is the process of building a bridge between the "smoking trance" which the client once enthusiastically embraced as a teenager or young adult, and the "non-smoking trance" which the client consciously recognises as being more useful for the present and the future. This bridging experience has been described as "inspiration," "flow" or "peak experience". Because each individual has unique resources and experiences, this transformation happens in a way which is just right for each individual. As Erickson put it:

> "the hypnotic state is an experience that belongs to the subject, derives from the subject's own accumulated learnings and memories, not necessarily consciously recognised, but possible of manifestation in a special state of nonwaking awareness. Hence the hypnotic trance belongs only to the subject; the operator can do no more than learn how to proffer stimuli and suggestions to evoke responsive behavior based upon the subject's own experiential past."[4]

Chapter 3

Fundamentals for success in smoking cessation

Three keys to success in smoking cessation through hypnotherapy

1. You must communicate powerfully with the particular client in front of you and tailor the session to their unique model of the world.
2. You must maintain a continuous connection with the client's moment-to-moment experience.
3. You must effectively educate your client both to stop smoking and to remain a non-smoker for life.

To achieve such a result, you, the hypnotherapist, will have to demonstrate all your flexibility and knowledge. Putting the client into an hypnotic trance and telling them to become a non-smoker does not necessarily mean that they will become a non-smoker or know how to stay one. It is more than likely that they will simply walk out of the door and immediately light up a cigarette. Conversely, many people successfully stop smoking without seeing a hypnotherapist at all. In the 1950s, before the health problems relating to smoking were discovered, some 75 percent of adults smoked. Today only 27 percent smoke. So about half the country has stopped smoking.

How then have so many people successfully quit? Many mothers who have come to see me to stop smoking have told me that they quit smoking when they become pregnant because they "simply couldn't" smoke during pregnancy for the baby's sake. Yet shortly after the birth they reverted to smoking. Some of them have repeated this pattern in subsequent pregnancies. Other people have maybe moved house or moved to a new country and found they simply did not want to smoke any more. Some have had a powerful moment of decision in which they became non-smokers instantly. In some cases they had a shock when a relative died of lung cancer or a heart attack caused by smoking, at which point they stopped. In each case there has been a moment of transformation in which the person became a non-smoker without any great effort of willpower. Sometimes they report physical cravings for a couple of weeks as the body cleansed itself of the accumulated poison, but in others there was no physical sensation whatsoever. The hypnotherapist's task is to engineer such a moment of transformation for the client, and to provide the tools to ensure that they stay a non-smoker in every possible future situation.

An article in the *New Scientist* in 1992 reported that "Hypnosis is the most effective way of giving up smoking, according to the largest ever scientific comparison of ways of breaking the habit." The magazine reported on research done by scientists at Iowa University who studied the results of 600 studies of a total of nearly 72,000 people in Europe and the USA who had successfully quit smoking. They found that 30 percent of those ex-smokers had quit using hypnotherapy, compared with 25 percent from aversion therapy, 24 percent from acupuncture, 10 percent from nicotine gum, nine percent from books and mail order advice and only 6 percent from willpower[1]. That looks extremely good for hypnotherapists; you will find that research cited in many a hypnotherapist's publicity material.

Despite this, the officially approved way to quit the smoking habit is through nicotine replacement therapy (NRT) products: patches, inhalers, gums and lozenges. These aim to reduce the craving after a person quits smoking by putting into the body an ever-decreasing amount of nicotine, until the nicotine supply is stopped completely. These NRT products deal only with the physical aspects of smoking and do not claim to touch upon the psychological aspects. According to the Iowa University study, only 10 percent of people who had successfully quit had done so by nicotine gum.

The physiology of smoking

The physiological aspects of smoking are minor compared with the overriding psychological aspects. Laboratory rats, monkeys and other animals are often forced to smoke thousands of cigarettes in scientific studies. Yet when a lit cigarette is placed where they could smoke it if they wanted, but they are not forced to do so, they do not make any move to smoke it, no matter how many cigarettes they have previously smoked.

Nevertheless, the human body undergoes a considerable shift when either starting smoking or giving it up. In most cases, when a person smokes their first cigarette, there is considerable discomfort. The body resists. The person feels dizzy, wants to be sick, sometimes actually does vomit, and coughs violently. The eyes water and the person might even turn green. That is usually what happens. However, with a minority of smokers, these physical manifestations do not take place at all. They take to smoking like a duck to water. The person enters such a state of rapture in the enthusiasm to become a smoker that the body's natural defence mechanisms are overridden in order to make the transition to the smoking life all the easier. In trance states, the human body exhibits a remarkable power to transcend experiences of pain and discomfort.

The person enters a state where the body "knows" unconsciously that smoking is so wonderful that the body accepts it without complaint.

If it is possible to override such physical sensations when the person *starts* smoking, then it is equally possible to do the same thing when they quit the habit. The hypnotherapist's job is to induce a similarly ecstatic state in which the unconscious communicates to the body that it is time to become a non-smoker and to enjoy all the benefits that derive from that.

Another physiological factor to bear in mind is what is called the "nicotine trick"[2]. By chance, it happens that the chemical effect of nicotine on the body is very similar to the experience of fear and anxiety. The first cigarette a person ever smokes produces a delayed feeling of physical tension in the body from inhaling the nicotine. It takes some minutes after finishing that first cigarette for the person to experience that feeling of physical tension. The physical tension causes the chest, face muscles and diaphragm to tighten slightly. That familiar feeling of tension is often labelled as a withdrawal symptom.

Now that feeling of tension is very similar to the physical experience of fear. When you experience fear, you also get that physical tension in the chest, face and diaphragm. Many young people smoke just one cigarette, experience that tension, and say, "Hey, I don't like this, I'm not going to smoke any more of those." So that feeling of tension disappears over the course of four days as the nicotine leaves the body. That youngster who smokes only one cigarette remains a non-smoker. However, other young people feel that sensation of tension after the first cigarette, assume that it is a feeling of fear, and then smoke a second cigarette in order to relieve what seems to be that feeling of fear. This simply starts the process all over again. It "resets" the body back to the beginning. That second cigarette recreates that delayed feeling of tension, so the person reaches for a third cigarette to relieve the feeling, then a fourth cigarette to relieve that, and so on. This is what is called "the nicotine trick": the smoker is tricked into believing that the delayed feeling of tension is in fact a feeling of fear. So the smoker keeps lighting up cigarette after cigarette in an attempt to relieve that feeling of fear – until the day that they stop. Once the person reaches the point where they simply let the nicotine leave the body, and do not smoke for the four days it takes for that to happen, then the body restores itself to that feeling of calm, health and well-being it enjoyed before the person started smoking. Thus the nicotine trick is beaten.

The power of intent

Hypnotherapy is holistic in the sense that in the course of a hypnosis session the client changes at an identity level. Rather than simply treating the symptoms – the unwanted behaviours – hypnotherapy for smoking is designed to fundamentally alter the way the person understands who they are. This is why I use the term "being a non-smoker" in preference to "not smoking".

The effective use of hypnotherapy for smoking cessation differs fundamentally from the standard prescription of nicotine replacement therapies such as patches, inhalers, gums and lozenges, or drugs such as Zyban (bupropion) or Champix (varenicline). With these, every smoker receives one standard product. It is assumed that enabling a person to quit smoking is primarily a question of changing chemical reactions inside the body.

In providing these products, the doctor or pharmacist takes an objective attitude: it might work, or it might not. Either way, according to that model, its effect is independent of the intent of the person providing the product.

With hypnotherapy, by contrast, the power of the therapist's intent is vital. The hypnotherapist must always be certain that the client will become a non-smoker. Therefore, assume success in advance, and communicate in a way that is congruent with that assumption. Even when talking to a potential client on the telephone before the session, if the client expresses any doubt or scepticism about the process, it is vital to reframe their negativity by saying something like:

> "You've already achieved success in many areas of life. You already know that once you assume that you can do something, it becomes a reality. When people assume that they will play well at sport, or pass an exam, or master a musical instrument, or learn to drive, they open a pathway which makes it happen. In the same way, once you believe that you will become a non-smoker, your mind and body do what is necessary to make that happen."

It is vital to challenge and refute any doubts that the client may express.

Focus on the positive

The effective hypnotherapist recognises that the client who intends to stop smoking is already a success, a winner, an achiever. Convey this message to them before, during and after the session, both explicitly and implicitly. When a sense of success, winning and achievement in one area of life is built up, it tends to set off a chain reaction which brings positive benefits in other areas. This is true not only of the individual's personal achievements, but also of those institutions to which the individual is emotionally attached. Studies of the output of factories in Britain found that productivity dramatically increased in the working days immediately after the local football team won a match. The successful performance of the local football club gave its supporters a boost which led to improved performance at their jobs.

In a similar way, the hypnotherapist seeks to praise the client's previous personal achievements, when they have tapped into resourcefulness to achieve some goal. This generalises, so that the client, at an unconscious level, is able to solve the smoking problem in the same resourceful way. An empowered, positive, motivated client, aware of their own resourcefulness and ability, finds the process of quitting smoking remarkably easy. In this business, flattery will get you everywhere!

Totally repudiate the attitude of "Let's hope for the best and see what happens." Convey certainty to your client in verbal and non-verbal communication, and it becomes infectious. Once the client catches that certainty and knows that they are becoming a non-smoker, it becomes a self-fulfilling prophecy.

Learning at an unconscious level

At any given moment the conscious mind is aware of only a very limited amount of information. Everything else is unconscious – including all our memories, our habits, our beliefs and our representations of the future. There is usually no useful reason to be consciously aware of everything happening in the body – the heartbeat, the circulation of blood, the immune system, the digestion of food, and thousands of other functions – otherwise you would not be able to do anything else! Therefore it makes sense for these functions to be coordinated by the inner intelligence of the unconscious mind.

It is useful to think of the unconscious mind as seeking to protect the person. When a person adopts the smoking habit, the unconscious regards that habit as the best, most immediately available way of helping that person *at that time*. The hypnotherapist's task is to assist the client's unconscious mind in finding a new, better way of achieving that positive intention than through smoking. We have to find the way to communicate with the client's unconscious mind to bring about this new solution.

The unconscious mind is creative in that it constantly forms new associations, learns, and helps the person move forward. The associations formed with the smoking habit when the person starts smoking as a teenager – or young adult – change with passage of time. As the smoker moves through life, so the need to prove membership of a particular group, rebel against authority or appear to be grown up, disappears. But the smoking habit remains. Unconsciously, these teenage – or young adult – associations are replaced by new ones: the cigarette becomes a crutch, a companion, a friend, a comfort, a means of introspection or of dealing with stress. In short, the unconscious mind forms new associations in relation to smoking anyway. Your task as a hypnotherapist is to facilitate, or guide, that process of the formation of new associations. You must enable the person to form new, more useful ways of gaining emotional support, introspection, stress relief and so on than through smoking.

An experience of fascination

The central aim of an hypnotic induction is to absorb the client in an experience of fascination. Clients often have an interest, hobby, sport or other enthusiasm which can be utilised. Find the activity which they enjoy doing for hour after hour and which absorbs all their attention. This might include gardening, painting, golf, yoga or any number of others. It simply depends on what the individual client enjoys. Ask the client to remember their greatest achievement with this activity: the flowers that gave the most pleasure in the garden, the watercolour they enjoyed painting the most, the lowest score at golf, the most satisfactory yoga session, or whatever it might be. Use this experience to lead to memories of achievement in other areas of life: perhaps their career, raising a family, learning to drive, recovering from ill-health, or achieving freedom from other unwanted habits such as alcoholism or nail-biting – whatever the client has experienced. Then ask the client's unconscious mind to draw an analogy by applying that same ability to create success to the process of becoming a non-smoker.

Many clients will have had experience of some system of personal development. Utilise this if the client tells you about it. One of my clients who wanted to stop smoking had been a kung fu champion and was now managing a pub. From the look of him, it was unlikely that he had any problems enforcing drinking-up time. After the first session he reverted to smoking. When he returned for a follow-up, he said that financial problems had been preying on his mind, and that these had caused him to go back to the habit. I asked him to remember his training in kung fu, which seeks to build up *chi* (universal life energy) and direct it under the kung fu master's control. I asked him to imagine that the financial problems were turning into opposing kung fu fighters, and that he had the task of defeating them through superior control of chi and fighting skill. After he imagined that experience, we went on to direct the chi in such a way as to clear out the smoking habit through the meridians of the body – a concept from traditional Chinese medicine, which has the same philosophy as kung fu. Because these concepts were real and powerful to the client, he was able to draw on his experience and beliefs, and thus use these resources to both stop smoking and solve his financial problems.

The same principle applies with any belief system in which the client participates. I have asked some clients to tap into their memories of spiritual experiences in order to pray to achieve their goals, to imagine a computer program controlling a robot which creates the desired outcome, and to visualise a tarot card reading or a horoscope being cast which predicts the result they are seeking. It all depends on the individual client's interests and experiences, and it is the therapist's job to communicate in terms which make sense to the client. The therapist's personal opinions, preferences or interests are irrelevant. As Erickson put it, "You never try to discredit what the patient knows is a reality for him."[3]

Ask yourself: what resources does this client have, and how can they be applied to enable them to become a non-smoker? All clients can be helped to tap into their creativity. I have asked clients to imagine dancing a ballet, creating a television commercial, writing a story, painting a picture, acting in a play or composing a piece of music that describes the process of becoming a non-smoker. Because the client enjoys this activity and can relate to it, the process is simple from their point of view. Music is particularly powerful, even among people who are not musicians. When you ask a client to recall a positive memory of being a non-smoker, you can add, "And perhaps there's some piece of music that you find inspiring, and maybe you can hear that music now as an accompaniment to this scene." If the client does internally hear their piece of music, it adds power to the technique; if not, rapport is maintained, because the words "perhaps" and "maybe" validate either experience.

The more the therapist is in harmony with the client's model of the world, the more effective the therapy will be.

Gaining control of immediate experience

Most clients find no difficulty in stopping smoking for the duration of the hypnotherapy session. That's no big deal. The issue here is what happens after the session. Are they going to be able to stay a non smoker in every situation for the rest of their lives? This is the real challenge, and this is where the therapist's influence is required. If the client already knew exactly how to make the changes on their own, presumably they would have already done so.

The hypnotherapist is able to influence the client because they listen closely to them, observe everything about them, and then tailor their communication towards that client's unique situation. At each stage of the session the therapist asks questions such as, "Can you tell me what you just experienced?" and "What are you aware of now?", to make sure that the desired result has been achieved. The therapist only ends the session when they are aware, as far as it is possible to be so, that the client has taken on the identity of a non-smoker.

After the client leaves the therapist's premises, they will inevitably be exposed to influences which are just as hypnotic as anything that was experienced during the session. The ex-smoker is likely to experience at least one of the following testing situations: socialising and drinking with smokers, living with a smoker, workplace stress, unexpected problems, physical cravings and the challenge of staying slim as a non-smoker. In any such challenging situation, the client must be able to overcome any temptation to smoke a cigarette. The client must know how to gain control over their subjective experience in the moment and make immediate changes to enable them to stay a non-smoker. The client must be proactive, participate fully in the process of achieving freedom from smoking, and be committed to staying that way permanently. If an individual who has been to see a hypnotherapist says something like, "It didn't work. I lit up half an hour after the session," then in that case the "hypnotherapy" was not performed adequately or effectively.

The client should be actively engaged in the process of change. They should never think of themselves as being passive recipients of the therapist's words, trusting to luck as to whether or not success is achieved. During their time with the hypnotherapist, the client learns how to challenge, deflect and redirect random thoughts and impulses in a way consistent with good health. In order to help them stay a non-smoker when the temptation to smoke arises – whether half an hour or five years after the session – I give the client a handout with these techniques written down and also recorded on a self-hypnosis CD.

Neuro-linguistic programming

There is nothing new under the sun. The techniques for mental control which have proven to be simplest, quickest and most effective for clients to make a change to their experience have been around for millennia. My background includes the study of NLP (neuro-linguistic programming) and I use NLP techniques in my hypnotherapy.

Neuro-linguistic programming is the system developed by Richard Bandler and John Grinder which aims to describe the structure of subjective experiences and enable changes to be made to those experiences quickly and easily. Bandler and Grinder studied the techniques of leading psychotherapists Milton Erickson, Fritz Perls and Virginia Satir and "modelled" what they did in therapy by systematising the elements that made their communications particularly effective.

One NLP technique used here in order to educate clients in gaining control over their experience is changing the *submodalities* of their experience. There are five *modalities* or senses: visual (V), auditory (A), kinesthetic (K), olfactory (O) and gustatory (G). Any subjective internal experience we become aware of within those modalities has *submodalities* – qualities or characteristics which vary across a range, and which we can adjust with our conscious mind. In practical hypnotherapy we deal mainly with the main three modalities: visual, auditory and kinesthetic. Submodalities are defined as "the special sensory qualities perceived by each of the senses". Using this method, the individual who experiences an impulse to smoke becomes aware of *how* that impulse is experienced. It could be in the form of a feeling, a sound or a voice, or seeing other people smoking, or less commonly a mental picture, or sometimes a taste or smell. Or it could be a combination of two or more of these. What makes the difference, subjectively, is the particular combination of sensory qualities of the experience. For example, the emotional impact of a film depends partly on the nature of the image – black and white or colour, brightly lit or shadowy, focused or fuzzy, and so on. These factors, as with the particular qualities of your mental images – the submodalities – can be changed, just by choosing to make them different. You are the director of your own mental movies.

Therefore, devote just as much attention to teaching the client methods of gaining control over their subjective experience in those situations when they become aware of the impulse to smoke. They can change the way they experience that by adjusting its submodalities. In the case of a feeling, that means such factors as the location, size, weight, movement and temperature. With a sound or voice, the submodalities include the location, volume, speed and tone. With a picture, they include size, focus, lighting, whether it is colour or black and white, and whether still or moving. By systematically altering the various qualities of an experience, the client can identify which of those submodalities have the greatest influence on the desire to smoke. Then, for example, by changing a key factor – making a pressure lighter, or further away – the client can quickly adjust their experience and realise that the desire has now disappeared. The client gains both knowledge of how to stay a non-smoker and a sense of self-mastery, and this has a knock-on effect on other aspects of the therapy.

Self-hypnosis

It is essential to teach every smoking-cessation client a method of self-hypnosis so that they know how to continue the work after the session, if need be. This can be understood as reminding the client that they already know how to hypnotise themselves, but need guidance in how to do it effectively and on demand. Self-hypnosis enables the individual to clear the mind, physically relax the body and enter a creative state in which positive suggestions can be made to the unconscious mind.

In the 1920s, the pharmacist Emile Coué published his book *Self Mastery Through Conscious Autosuggestion*. His technique was simple. He would have a person focus the conscious mind on the task of moving the fingers along a piece of string with twenty knots on it, like a rosary, while repeating the suggestion, "Every day in every way, I am getting better and better." Since then, countless methods of self-hypnosis have been developed. The one presented in this book is as simple as possible, so that every client can do it easily. Once your client knows how to change state at will, and make suggestions to the unconscious mind, they are no longer a slave to random impulses and are able to direct the course of their own life.

Getting it right at every stage

Effective hypnotherapy, particularly with smoking cessation, depends on getting it right at every stage in the session. The smoker – even one who consciously wants to quit – may latch on to any excuse, however absurd, to cling on to the habit, or, having stopped, to revert to it in some situation in daily life. Any aspect of the therapy which fails to connect with the client's experience, or which the client might interpret as "giving permission" to stay smoking, is likely to end up with them sticking with the habit.

Imagine the hull of a ship with a tiny hole in it. That hull could be constructed of the most resilient, waterproof material known to shipbuilding, but the water would still flood the ship through that hole as surely as if the entire hull were made of newspaper.

If the client chooses to disregard your preparation and revert to smoking in some situation which you prepared them for, then that is the client's responsibility, not yours.

Put yourself into the most empowered state possible

Although during hypnosis most of the attention is placed on the state of the client, bear in mind that the hypnotist's state is equally important. It is recommended that before you do any work with a client, you use self-hypnosis or some other technique to put yourself into the most resourceful state possible. Create positive optimism and belief that the client will become a non-smoker. Observe the client, listen closely to what they say, and respond powerfully to what you hear and see. Get in touch with the vast knowledge of hypnotic and allied techniques in your unconscious mind, so that what you need springs out spontaneously when required. Banish any thoughts about issues in your own life which are currently on your mind, at least for the duration of your session with the client. Give your client 100 percent of your dedicated effort and attention.

In order to achieve that empowered state, prepare a self-hypnosis routine which you use every day before seeing clients. Effective hypnotherapy can be exhausting for the therapist, both mentally and physically, but it is a satisfying sense of exhaustion when the energy has been directed productively. You also need a means of snapping out of the powerful state you have built up for therapy once the session ends. This could be physical exercise, listening to music, engaging with some hobby, or having a drink in congenial company. Whatever your preferred method, find a reliable way to come down from the energised state which you use for hypnotherapy.

Use common sense

Hypnotherapy is most effective when it is grounded in the concrete realities of the client's experience. Although you have a vast range of techniques at your disposal, don't get caught up in a technique and forget common sense. All the "tricks" of hypnosis – ideomotor response, catalepsy, amnesia, hypermnesia, dissociation, time distortion, spontaneous anaesthesia, future-pacing and so on are fancy names for human faculties which we have each experienced countless times. These ways of manipulating experience are means to an end, not ends in themselves. If the client isn't getting a particular technique, move on. Keep the flow and energy of the session at a high level. If an idea pops into your mind which you think can help this particular client in this particular session, then express that idea to the client – regardless of whether it is "hypnotic" or not. The client may experience a moment of insight, breakthrough or transformation from that idea which helps them become a non-smoker. You are a unique, resourceful and creative individual – and so is your client.

Positively welcome "difficult" clients

A proverb says, "Calm seas never made good sailors." In order to become an effective and resourceful seafarer, it is not enough merely to read a couple of textbooks and then steer your boat across a tranquil stretch of water with high visibility on a sunny day. To become truly skilled, you have to successfully guide your boat through high storms in sub-zero temperatures in the blackest night in winter, through waves rising higher than your mast, and with gale-force winds, freezing rain and bolts of lightning striking your vessel. Then you can call yourself a navigator.

It is with the more "difficult" or "awkward" clients that you achieve mastery in hypnotherapy. It is easy enough when a client who attends for smoking cessation is an amiable and cooperative sort of person, introspective and creative, perhaps experienced in meditation, who masters the techniques instantly, goes into deep trance as soon as you suggest it, becomes a non-smoker immediately, pays the fee, and stays a non-smoker for life.

However, most clients are not like that. Some think that they are perpetual smokers who can't quit. Others are rude, hostile and uncooperative. Some express resentment of the therapist for seeking to deprive them of their little treat. Others find it difficult to connect with the techniques used. Others will blame the therapist for the fact that they continue to smoke after the session. A few will try and evade payment, one way or another. Almost certainly, you will encounter all these types, and more.

I recommend that you positively welcome working with these difficult clients. They will stretch your communicational abilities to the limit, and beyond, and inspire you to adapt the techniques you know and create new ones. They should also encourage you to study therapeutic techniques further to find ways of handling such individuals. You will learn far more from working with these difficult clients than from the relatively straightforward ones. Easy clients never make skilled hypnotherapists.

The context of hypnotherapy

Both money and power significantly influence the nature of the hypnotherapy session, depending upon the context. When a medical practitioner, dentist or chartered psychologist uses hypnosis with patients, this is usually provided within the context of a government health service paid for by taxation, or by a private insurance scheme for which either the patient or their employer has paid. In either context, the patient is not paying directly for the session from their own pocket. As a result, the therapy can continue across multiple sessions with no additional cost to the patient. Also, doctors and dentists – less so psychologists – are *ex officio* authority figures whose status enables them to tell their patients what to do. The very fact that such a professional is telling the patient to stop smoking, or achieve some other goal, means that the patient attributes high value to it, and that makes the therapy more effective.

With a so-called "lay" hypnotherapist, the dynamics are completely different. A hypnotherapist has to communicate with the client as an equal in every respect. The balance of power shifts over the course of the session. If the session is successful, power tends to be transferred from the therapist to the client over its course. In fact, the client is really in a position of power because they are paying for the session. Almost always, the question of whether the session is worth the money will be playing in the client's mind before, during and possibly after the session. Although they might not say it aloud, it will be on their minds. You have to impress them with what they experience very quickly indeed. This is precisely why NLP submodalities, self-hypnosis and cognitive self-talk – which demonstrate that the power lies with the client – are taught early in the session. As the client realises how quickly subjective experiences can be changed, they are likely to accept that value for money is being achieved. While the client might consider these techniques to be merely "common sense" when the therapist demonstrates them, the point is that the client is now taking action to become a non-smoker, and has acquired the power to cease to be a slave of random impulses.

It is essential to explain everything in terms the client understands. No client will do something simply because a lay hypnotherapist tells them to. It is equally important to aim to achieve the desired result in a single session, offering back-up if the client requires it. Clients are not going to keep coming back for session after session, paying money every time without having achieved the result they desire. So do it in one session.

In hundreds of books on hypnosis I have read or looked through, there has never been a single mention of the vital yet somehow "indelicate" subject of the financial context in which hypnosis takes place. Yet for many clients, this is an important consideration, and you have to ensure that you deal with it. In the early days of my practice, one client who attended for smoking cessation sat down and his very first words were, "Seventy-five quid, mate," as if challenging me to prove that the session was worth that price. You have to convince the client by word and action that they are getting full value for the fee. One way of doing this is to build momentum in the session and keep the pace as fast and powerful as the client can handle.

The role of the hypnotherapist

Treat the client as though they are in charge! All that the hypnotherapist can do is pace and lead. Pacing means connecting with the client's experience in the moment. Leading means guiding the client towards achieving the solution the client is seeking. The therapist is tapping into and launching the client's innate creative learning abilities so that the client becomes a non-smoker. It is equally important that the hypnotherapist educates the client to sail the stormy seas of life, so that they always have a more useful response to every possible future situation than reaching for a cigarette.

Here are insights on the nature of hypnotherapeutic learning from the two doctors of medicine who founded the American Society of Clinical Hypnosis. In 1948, Milton Erickson wrote:

> "The induction and maintenance of a trance serve to provide a special psychological state in which patients can re-associate and reorganize their inner psychological complexities and utilize their own capacities in a manner in accord with their own experiential life. … It is this experience of re-associating and reorganizing his own experiential life that eventuates in a cure, not the manifestation of responsive behavior, which can, at best, satisfy only the observer. … In other words, hypnotic hypnotherapy is a learning process for the patient, a process of reeducation. Effective results in hypnotic psychotherapy,

or hypnotherapy, derive only from the patient's activities. The therapist merely stimulates the patient into activity, often not knowing what that activity may be. ... Such reeducation is, of course, necessarily in terms of the patient's life experiences, his understandings, memories, attitudes, and ideas; it cannot be in terms of the therapist's ideas and opinions."[4]

In an interview in 1987, William Kroger said of hypnosis that:

"It's simply a state of increased awareness. If you're more aware, whatever you hear is going to sink in better. If it sinks in better, you get better responses, whether it's hitting a golf ball or having an erection. ... I have been studying hypnosis for more than 60 years and it's not complicated at all. It's a very simple process of everyday life. Hypnosis is merely a process of getting a message through without redundancy. ... Minimizing the signal-to-noise ratio ... hypnosis is nothing more or less than the transmission of a message in a minimum noise environment. That's all! Why do we have to have all these other damn meanings to it? They obfuscate everything!"[5]

Those two quotations summarise two different ways of looking at the same phenomenon.

Erickson emphasises that the transformation which takes place in hypnotherapy is a process of internal reorganisation of the client's experience, and that the therapist's task is to facilitate that inner restructuring. Everything happens inside the client's unconscious mind. The hypnotherapist can only work with the existing resources within the client's unconscious. The client must become the captain of their own destiny, running a tight ship, setting the course and directing the various crew members in their various and interlocking roles.

Kroger emphasises that effective hypnotic communication means getting the therapeutic message across to the client without interference or "noise". Noise includes: the constant running commentary going on in the client's mind – which is often cynical and sceptical; saying things that the client does not agree with or does not understand; the client being distracted; or the therapist saying things that do not connect with the client's model of the world.

The smoking issue differs significantly from all other issues with which hypnotherapists deal. With smoking cessation, the hypnotherapist's task is to communicate powerfully and unambiguously with the client that they are to stop smoking and stay stopped. Whatever else may happen, achieving that outcome is essential. With other issues in hypnotherapy, the final desired outcome is uncertain. With weight control, for example, the "correct" eating habits and weight for one person are not necessarily appropriate for another. Indeed, in some cases, such as anorexics, losing any more weight could be dangerous or even fatal. In order to be effective with weight control, you have to find out what solution is most appropriate for that particular client and use techniques to achieve it. With the issue of building confidence, you have to learn what confidence means to a particular client, in what situations it is required, and how to draw on the client's internal resources in order to create it. With the issue of emotional change, there could be many possible ways of helping a client forward to a variety of different possible outcomes, in each of which they would feel happier.

With smoking there is only one acceptable outcome. Whatever else may happen, and by whatever route you get there, the client must stop smoking and stay stopped. I recall a conversation with a Gestalt psychotherapist. He said that if a client were to come to him with a view to stopping smoking, he would facilitate a dialogue between that part of the client which wanted to stop smoking and that part which wanted to stick with the smoking habit. If the part which wanted to stay smoking won that argument, then the session would end with a decision that the client should stay a smoker.

Some hypnotherapists, too, may take the view that the purpose of the hypnotherapy session is for the client to understand their own situation and to make an informed decision about what they want to do. You might take the view that if the client learns that it is not appropriate at this time – that the benefits of the smoking outweigh the possible benefits later of becoming a non-smoker – then it seems reasonable to respect their choice, and invite them back when their circumstances change.

With all due respect to such therapists, I take a different approach. It is true that every client who attends for any kind of treatment for smoking cessation does indeed have two conflicting parts: the part that is still smoking and the part that wants to quit. My own view is the hypnotherapist's task is to presuppose the outcome of being a non-smoker, to actively take the side of the part that wants to quit, and to induce the part that is clinging to smoking to find a more useful way of achieving its positive intention. The risk is that if the therapist takes a "neutral" role, as if refereeing between the two parts, then the smoking part is often likely to win. This is partly through inertia and partly because of "smoker's logic" which rationalises everything – whatever the smoker experiences – in a way favourable to staying smoking. My view is that the hypnotherapist should always be biased in favour of the part that wants to quit, no matter what.

However, some clients do manage to drastically reduce their cigarette consumption, say, from twenty a day down to two, and regard that as a personal success with which they are happy. Now the central drawback of such a reduction is that it is confusing for the body. Many who reduce their intake in that way find their cigarette consumption gradually drifting upwards again until they are back on twenty a day. Certainly you can point that out to clients, and encourage them to set the goal of quitting smoking completely. However, the hypnotherapist's role is to assist the client in achieving *the client's* personal goals, not those of some outside authority. With clients who are content with a reduction in smoking, accept that as a success by the client's criteria.

The hypnotherapist's communicational style

During the hypnotherapy session, the hypnotherapist is communicating with the continuous flow of the client's subjective experience, seeking to guide that experience towards the desired goal (such as becoming a non-smoker). One of the most effective ways of communicating effectively is to tell stories. Some of the stories I use have a "scientific" basis, as that gives them more credibility. In order to make a point stick in the client's mind, I may refer to some alleged scientific research which has "proved" something or other, even though a scientist might regard my account as an over-simplification, an exaggeration, a half-truth or an urban myth.

For example, many clients say that they are concerned about the possibility of losing control of their actions while drinking alcohol, and reverting to smoking in that situation. With such clients, I tell them the story of a psychological experiment in which one group of subjects was given a non-alcoholic drink which they were told contained alcohol, while another group were given a drink which they were told was alcoholic but which contained no alcohol. An hour later the subjects who believed that they had consumed alcohol were "acting drunk", while there was no observable difference in the behaviour of the other group. Now I had read about this experiment somewhere, without making a note of the reference, and had always assumed that it was true. However, I have not been able to find any reference to this experiment in the psychological literature. It may well be an urban myth, or a misunderstanding, over-simplification or exaggeration of an actual experiment that did take place somewhere at some time. It could even have been a hoax perpetrated by some prankster. So is there a problem here? Many of my clients have been impressed by the account of the experiment, and it has helped them stay non-smokers while continuing to enjoy drinking. My view is that it is more effective to tell the client a convincing story or cite an urban myth – apocryphal as it may be – than for me to simply say, "Oh, but you *can* stay in control of your actions even after a few drinks."[6]

The lay hypnotherapist is not – at least in the context of therapy – engaged in scientific education. They are engaged in communicating in such a way as to produce the desired effect on the particular client. One of my smoking cessation clients was a lady from Belize, who was of Central American Indian origin. Early in the session, she showed me an amulet which she wore as a means of protecting her spirit from any evil influences that might have tried to enter during hypnotic trance. I immediately replied, in a matter-of-fact tone of voice, that we were going to use that the spiritual power of that amulet in order to chase away the "smoking spirit" and replace it with healthy and protective spirits. This is the sort of terminology in which Central American Indian shamans and healers communicate. The session then continued largely in those terms, and the client became a non-smoker.

If the client comes to you with any preconceptions about hypnosis, it is usually best to work with them rather than try to "correct" them. The hypnotherapist Jerry Valley has an impressive-looking pendulum on prominent display in his consulting room. Sometimes he will deal with a client who says something like, "A pendulum. I've heard that when you focus your attention on that for one minute, you go into a really deep trance." Valley replies, "That's right," and proceeds to remove the pendulum from its display and use it as an object of fixation. Other clients say something like, "A pendulum? You're not going to try and hypnotise me with any of that hoary old nonsense, are you?" Valley replies, "Oh, no, that's just for show. It's an antique. We use much more modern methods these days."

The less mental "work" the client has to do, the better. The meaning of the communication is the response you get.

Fundamentals

In summary, then, you need to pay attention to …

- The therapist's state. Make sure that your own state is optimised to be as resourceful as possible. See Chapter 4.
- The client's expectations. Do as much as you can to maximise the client's expectations for success, both before and during the session. See Chapter 4.
- The first encounter – on the phone and in the office. See Chapters 4 and 5.
- The rest of the client's life, by educating them how to stay a non-smoker permanently. See Chapter 6.
- Communicating effectively with the client's unconscious – and checking your work. See Chapter 7.

You might like to consider which direction you want to move towards in your career as a hypnotherapist dealing with smoking cessation, beyond doing one-to-one therapy. Two avenues discussed later are:

- Running smoking cessation groups open to the public. See Chapter 13.
- Offering smoking cessation seminars to the corporate market. See Chapter 14.

As a hypnotherapist, you may well already be familiar with many of the concepts and techniques included in this volume. Some are my own innovations, while others have simplified, combined or adapted the techniques of others. Everything here is based on what I have done in the real world, and has been tested for its effectiveness with clients.

Every client is different. For hypnotherapy to be effective, you will need to adjust the process to meet the needs and the beliefs of the individual client and situation. What you say and what you do have to make sense to that unique individual sitting in front of you. *You* have to be flexible in your approach. Do whatever it takes to achieve success; neither you nor the client should be satisfied with a negative result.

When I am with a client, we will keep working, if necessary, using new and different approaches, until the outcome is achieved. Hold in mind the thought: "my client is here to teach me." Look on any obstacles a particular client faces as challenges which inspire you to further study of techniques for personal development, not necessarily from hypnotherapy, which might be useful in helping this particular client move forward. Indeed, tap into your creativity, innovate new techniques, get good results with them – and then teach them to other therapists through articles, lectures, seminars and perhaps your own book. Hypnotherapy never stands still; why not make your own unique contribution to its development?

Chapter 4

Preparing for the session

Careful planning gives maximum prospect for success

Success in hypnotherapy, particularly with smoking cessation, depends on getting a large number of small details right, first time, every time. The more meticulously you prepare for your client in advance, the more effective the session is likely to be.

Before every commercial flight, the pilots go through a written checklist with one another. They confirm that every instrument is functioning and set correctly before they are cleared for take-off. Even if they know the checklist by heart, and have been flying for decades, they go through the entire list every time. Pilots have responsibility for their passengers' lives. They could probably get away with relying on memory for their pre-flight checks most of time. But it is a statistical certainty that sooner or later, with millions of flights worldwide, human error would creep in, tiny things would go wrong, and preventable air disasters would happen.

Hypnotherapists, too, are responsible for ensuring that every element of the client's experience is optimised for success. Particularly with smoking cessation, what we do can make the difference between life and death for the client. According to the US Surgeon General's report on smoking in 2004, a man who successfully quits smoking adds an average of 13.2 years to his life, a woman 14.5 years. Because the client's state is affected by a multitude of factors, not just those classified as "hypnotic" or "therapeutic", you want to be certain that each of those factors is orientated towards the desired outcome.

There is a huge literature for therapists about how to use hypnosis, NLP, cognitive therapy and other approaches. While much of it contains useful information about how to deal with clients when they actually arrive and are sitting in front of the therapist, there is relatively little on how to prepare for the session in advance in order to maximise the possibilities for success.

The overall context of the therapy, including the client's prior assumptions about it, and the state they are in on arrival at the therapist's premises, can be just as significant as anything that happens during the actual session – and probably more so. It is frequently said that the effectiveness of a hypnotherapy session does not begin merely when the client goes into a formal hypnotic trance, but as soon as the client sits down in front of the therapist. In fact the effectiveness of the session starts long before the client actually meets the therapist.

Positively influencing the client before the session

Hypnotherapy is all about influencing the client's state. "State" refers to the combination of physiological, emotional and cognitive factors that a person experiences in the moment. When the client arrives at your premises, you want them to be in as calm, resourceful and optimistic a state as can reasonably be expected.

The hypnotherapist has a responsibility to take meticulous care to optimise the client's state from the moment the client even hears about what the therapist can do, right through to the months and years after the session, as the client deals with life as a non-smoker. This process starts with the hypnotherapist's reputation for getting successful results. If a potential client who wants to stop smoking has seen a friend, relative or colleague successfully and easily become a non-smoker after a session with you, and they book a session, then already that new client's state of expectation is a positive resource that matches anything you could possibly achieve in the session itself.

Expectations tend to be realised. People tend to relate what they see and hear other people do to themselves. This is an automatic process, not requiring any conscious effort. Clients who book as a result of the transformation they have seen in someone else have already built up an expectation of becoming non-smokers. The very process of predicting a successful outcome tends to bring about that outcome – *if the prediction is believed by the person hearing it.*

You are also in a strong position with those clients who attend after having heard you give a talk or demonstration about hypnosis. People respond to people. When they hear you explain how hypnosis can improve people's lives, see it demonstrated before their eyes, and maybe experience it in a group exercise, the whole process comes to life in their imagination. Definitely talk to people individually after the demonstration and leave leaflets on their seats so that they can contact you.

Similar strong expectations for success arise when the client has read a press article about you, an article you have yourself written for the press or a news-letter, or seen you on television or heard you on the radio. If something in these media appearances strikes a chord with the reader, listener or viewer, an expectation for success is built up and they will seek you out. Of course, this applies to every issue with which hypnotherapists deal, not just smoking.

On the other hand, that positive expectation will be nowhere near as strong if a potential client approaches you as a result of picking up one of your leaflets or reading an advertisement you have paid for, or finds you in a directory or on the Internet. Indeed, it is probable that such clients will be sceptical, hesitant, cynical and doubtful. They may book an appointment and fail to show up, without giving notice. Or they might suddenly call an hour or two before the session and cancel. Others, when they do turn up, will be hostile, critical and sometimes downright rude. A very small handful will try to evade payment after the session. They might give you a cheque that bounces, or use a credit card that shows up as invalid, or simply sprint out of the door without paying. This is what is known in the restaurant trade as "eat and run". In no such case do you have any legal redress against such clients. Virtually all such difficult clients come from leaflets, directories, paid advertising or the Internet. The good clients, who turn up more or less on time, have a positive and cooperative attitude, and who pay reliably, are the ones you get from the three referral sources mentioned above. In the long run, you want to have a practice built up predominantly of referral clients, rather than respondents to advertisements, leaflets or visits to a website.

Even with potential clients who do not know anyone whom you have helped, you can still influence them positively before you actually meet. If your publicity and any articles in the media about you are favourable to you and to hypnosis in general, then potential clients will approach you with a positive attitude, which will improve the prospects for success when the actual session takes place. Your aim with each of these media is to inform people in your community about what hypnotherapy is and how it can help them achieve goals which are important to them. There is no pressure being put on the potential client to make use of your services; people can choose to contact you or not. When they do, be prepared to answer questions, by telephone, letter or email, without obligation.

Once the enquirer telephones, you are in strong position to influence them positively. You can create in them a self-fulfilling prophecy by future-pacing a successful outcome. Both your words and the way you say them should display a calm and confident certainty in the achievement of the desired outcome. If the client simply wants to be sent information, then send a personal letter with your brochure. End the letter with the phrase "Always glad to help" and sign the letter in blue ink. It is a remarkable fact, known to the mail order industry for many decades, that a signature in blue ink dramatically increases the response to an offer. Many companies go to the expense of two-colour printing in their promotional material just to ensure that the signature is blue.

What to say when a potential client first calls

Potential clients who contact you about smoking cessation will have had different experiences and expectations. Most enquirers will be calling because they want to quit smoking themselves, although some will be contacting you on behalf of a partner or family member.

There are three things you need to do in the initial telephone conversation: to establish rapport, to ask questions and to encourage the client to make a booking.

Establishing rapport

Rapport is really about ensuring that non-verbal communication is as effective as possible. The essential elements of telephone rapport are matching the speed, volume, tone and modulation of the enquirer's voice. This enables the client to think of you – accurately enough – as someone who is "on their wavelength". However, avoid taking this to extremes, or the caller might think that you are mimicking or making fun of them.

The content of the conversation depends on what the client says. If the enquirer has been referred by a client whom you have already helped – whether with smoking cessation or some other issue – then you can ask how that other person is faring. You can be sure that that person has achieved a good result; that is precisely why the present enquirer is calling. Once the enquirer has given you a description, ask the enquirer to convey your congratulations and say in a matter-of-fact tone something like, "Yes, I knew Charlie could do it, it was simply a question of tapping into his inner ability to make it happen." Talk as if it was the simplest thing in the world. The enquirer is likely to assume that their own transformation will be just as simple and effective.

If the enquirer has been referred by a doctor, dentist, osteopath or other health professional, then take the opportunity to talk about how another client who was referred from the same source achieved a positive outcome (without mentioning the client's name, of course). This, too, helps to build a positive expectation for success.

If the enquirer has heard about you by picking up a leaflet, seeing an advertisement or finding you on the Internet, then they are likely to be more sceptical and to want considerably more information before committing. With such enquirers, you not only explain the process, but also ask questions about the client's experiences. You can then give an account of another client you have helped who has had similar experiences.

Asking questions

With those telephone enquirers who take the lead in the conversation by asking questions, you simply respond with informative answers. However, with those who are more reticent, you should take the lead by asking them courteous and non-intrusive questions about their experiences and what they are seeking. This may help them clarify their goals as well as giving you information about how you can best help them.

With enquirers who want to become non-smokers themselves, ask about their experience of smoking, whether they have stopped before, and if so by what method and for how long. If they have tried methods such as NRT products, group seminars or acupuncture, explain how hypnotherapy differs from them. Ask them whether they have encountered hypnotherapy before, and if so in what context. It is conceivable that they have visited a hypnotherapist before, but did not stop smoking, or else did stop for a while and reverted to the habit. If so, explain that what makes you different from many other hypnotherapists is that you emphasise the use of techniques to enable a client to stay a non-smoker permanently in every situation. Never denigrate another hypnotherapist or other smoking cessation methods.

You can explain that people smoke for a reason. While that may have been a valid reason when they were much younger, somehow those reasons have never been updated. You could ask them what role smoking plays in their life today. With the information the client gives, you can explain how hypnotherapy can enable them to find a new and more useful way of achieving the positive intention which smoking has played in their past and present.

A common question which telephone enquirers ask is, "What is your success rate?" Reply as follows:

> "In your case, 100 percent. (Pause.) The reason I say that is because with each individual it's going to be either zero percent – if they go back to smoking – or else 100 percent if they successfully become non-smokers. It's not a game of chance. The reality is that if you are choosing to become a non-smoker of your own free will, then it's a very straightforward process."

Putting it this way eliminates the idea that there is anything random or haphazard about hypnotherapy from the enquirer's mind. You could add:

> "The only people for whom it can be a little bit more tricky are those who are being frog-marched to me by someone else, maybe their partner, or their parents, or their doctor. For a person who has not come of their own free will, the idea of a success rate won't make sense, as that person is not ready yet to become a hypnotherapy client."

If the client presses you for a success rate, then continue:

> "But in general, bearing that in mind, x percent [whatever your actual "success rate" is] of people who come and see me become non-smokers. But in your particular case, if you're choosing to become a non-smoker for yourself, it's 100 percent."

Unless facing some urgent appointment, I will generally talk to the enquirer for as long as they want. I want to come across as a source of help and advice which people can call without obligation, risk or pressure.

Encouraging the enquirer to book

If the enquirer does not want to book immediately, then ask if you can send some information through the mail. It is more likely to be read and kept if sent by regular mail than by e-mail. If the enquirer has information about your services on paper, they are far more likely to book at some point in the future than if they have to depend on memory. It is extraordinary how long people will keep written publicity material. One client came to see me for smoking cessation in response to a particular leaflet of mine that was distributed *eleven years* previously.

However, if the client does not want to give these details and refuses a brochure, accept that, and simply say, "That's fine. Just call me any time I can be of help." High-pressure selling has no role to play in the promotion of hypnotherapy.

Remember that your intention is to get the enquirer to book a session. Once the person expresses the desire to book, ask, "Is there any particular day which suits you best?" Once they name a day, you can ask, "Would you prefer morning, afternoon or evening?" If the client says "Afternoon", then offer them a choice of, say, 1 pm and 4.30 pm. You are giving the impression – accurate or otherwise – of a full diary, and giving the client the *illusion of choice*. Book them in and then say, "Thank you. I'll send you an appointment card with a map. I'm sure you'll be able to find it." Avoid negatives such as, "You can't miss it." Remember that the unconscious has difficulty in processing a negative. The unconscious may well take such a phrase as an instruction for a negative hallucination – and they will miss it. It's more useful to give sensory information, such as what the building looks like, the colour of the door, and what else they will see by way of landmarks.

This approach is simple, explains everything in sufficient detail, and continues the process of pre-conditioning the client for a successful outcome. It is important to "guide" the client in this way. If the client gets the impression that you have absolutely no clients and can come at any time, this may well raise a question in their mind as to why that should be the case. By giving the impression that you are fairly busy, and suggesting a specific time, the client will be reassured that many others are availing themselves of your services. Whether that is true, of course, doesn't matter. You can rely on the *herd mentality* or *social proof* (to use the polite term).

Having made the booking, confirm it in writing. Send the client an appointment card with, for instance, "*Wednesday* 15th November" on it – because most people think in terms of days of the week, not dates of the month – and the time. Include a map which is easy to understand, and give details about car parking availability and the means of reaching you by public transport (if any). In addition, as part of the pre-framing process, write a letter on printed headed paper saying something like:

Dear Mr/Ms Blank,

Thank you for booking an appointment to stop smoking through hypnotherapy. Please find enclosed an appointment card giving the time and date. The fee will be £x.

When we meet, we will work on showing you how to use self-hypnosis to create calmness and resourcefulness in any situation, and we will also enable your unconscious mind to learn to live as a non-smoker.

In order to prepare yourself for the session, it is a good idea to imagine what life is going to be like in different situations – home life, socialising, your daily routine, travelling, and so on – once you become a non-smoker. Let yourself enjoy a pleasant fantasy or daydream about what it will be like.

If it becomes necessary to rearrange this appointment, please give at least 48 hours' notice, as this helps us with scheduling and is greatly appreciated.

Look forward to meeting you on the day.

With best wishes,

Yours sincerely,

[name]

If you are writing to a person's work address, then in order to protect their privacy, write the word "PERSONAL" on the front of the envelope. This ensures that it will be read only by the addressee.

The purpose of these preparations is to assure the client that they are being looked after, and to continue to pre-frame them for a successful outcome. It also increases the likelihood that the client will actually turn up for the appointment. This is partly because you have given a message about how they will benefit, and partly because it is less likely that they will misunderstand or forget. Including the map and details about parking and transport makes it easy for the client to find you; they are more likely to arrive on time, calm and relatively at ease. If the client has followed your advice and "daydreamed" about life as a non-smoker, then they may already be well on the way to becoming a non-smoker.

However, there will be occasions when a client does arrive late or flustered or both. Make sure that you leave gaps of at least half an hour between clients to allow for the possibility of late arrivals, or sessions overrunning their allotted time. These gaps also give you the chance to rest between clients. It is important to switch off from your previous client, especially after those sessions that did not go well, and to build up your energy and resourcefulness for the next client. You might like to use the brief self-hypnosis exercise later in this chapter, or develop your own, in order to do that.

If a client does arrive late, take it in your stride and do not mention it at the beginning at all. If the client gives an explanation or apology, accept it as if it is no big deal one way or the other. However, if and when that same client books a subsequent session, give a little gentle reminder that arriving punctually enables things to run smoothly, ensures that the client gets all the time they deserve, and is fair to subsequent clients. If a client arrives in a flustered state, then there is no need to make an issue out of it. Simply extend the period of rapport-building, if necessary, so that you lead the client's attention through small talk about some pleasant and interesting topic, and therefore away from whatever caused them to feel flustered. The client's state will alter along with this.

In my experience, the maximum number of one-to-one hypnotherapy clients one can comfortably deal with in a single day is four. Any more than that becomes too great a strain on the therapist. It is essential to give your clients as much of your "energy" as they need to achieve the transformation they are seeking. So plan your week such that the clients' appointments are spread out as far apart as is realistic.

Using self-hypnosis to optimise the therapist's state

The physical environment where the therapy takes place, whether a clinic of some sort or the therapist's home, must be spotless. If it is not, then the client may quickly turn against the entire process.

The hypnosis literature covers a great deal about the hypnotic subject's state: the hypnoid state, the light trance state, the medium state, the deep state, the somnambulistic state, the Esdaile state, and one hell of a state! What is not included in these books is how the client's state is affected by the overall context within which the hypnosis happens. If your client encounters something in the environment that they dislike, such as the bathroom being a mess, or the therapist wearing scruffy shoes or having unkempt hair, then that can affect them far more powerfully – and negatively – than any hypnotic technique which the therapist carries out. Therefore everything must be ready before the appointed time for the actual session. I have found that going through the checklist in Chapter 10 is an excellent way to ensure that everything in the environment is optimised for the client's positive state.

Another aspect of the hypnotherapeutic process which receives little attention in the books is the *therapist*'s state. The hypnotherapist should be in a peak state of resourcefulness, positivity and optimism. With regard to smoking cessation, the therapist must convey absolute certainty that the client is becoming a non-smoker. It is essential to be focused entirely on the client, so that every detail of their verbal and non-verbal communication is noticed – and, where appropriate, utilised. Effective hypnotherapists do not have off days. About twenty minutes before the client is due to arrive, clear your mind of any concerns which may have been weighing on it, and create an inner "zone of resourcefulness", so that you are at a peak of effectiveness. What follows is a self-hypnosis routine which enables you to do that.

A brief self-hypnosis exercise to prepare yourself for the session

You could either read the following words and go along with them, or record them in your own voice onto a computer or CD and play them to prepare yourself for the next client.

> "Breathing, slowly, deeply, and evenly. And, as you breathe in slowly, filling your lungs with air from the bottom to the top, and slowly expel all of that air, so that you are breathing completely new air, in and out, in an endless rhythm. Focusing your attention on the moments between the breaths, the moment where there is no breath.

> "And just be aware of the most relaxed part of your body now. And just imagine that that most relaxed part has a particular colour, the colour of relaxation. And just imagine that all the air you are breathing in is that same colour of relaxation. So that every time you breathe in, you are inhaling in that air which is the colour of relaxation. And every time you breathe out, so you're breathing out tension and stress and tiredness, and inhaling the air which is the colour of relaxation.

"So now focus your awareness on your tongue. Just imagine that there is a little slick of oil on the roof of your mouth, just at that point in the middle of the bridge above your front teeth. Now place the tip of your tongue at that exact point, and imagine that you are balancing that slick of oil, holding it in that position, so that your tongue becomes still. And notice how quiet your mind becomes as you do that."

The continuous "running commentary" in the conscious mind corresponds to tiny movements in the tongue, in which the tongue is "saying" the words of that monologue. If you stop the tongue from moving, so too that inner monologue ceases. This can be achieved by either physically holding the tongue with the thumb and forefinger, or by placing the tip of the tongue on the roof of the mouth, as described in the above paragraph.

"You are a highly capable hypnotherapist. You are a resourceful communicator. Your senses are sharp and your energy high. Your presence and skill guides your clients forward. Your clients gain measurable and specific improvements in their lives from coming to see you. You are successful, a winner, an achiever.

"So just see, in your mind's eye, how in this very room you are going to empower your next client to the best of your ability. Visualise yourself with that client, experiencing powerful rapport. Notice your own posture, expression, breathing. Listen to your own voice and the things you are saying. And be satisfied that you are performing as powerfully as you have ever performed. So that any time you want, you can step inside your own body in that picture, feel the way your body feels in this peak state, see your client and hear your own voice, and really notice the difference. Just take a few moments to experience that, to embrace your own power, and then, in your own time, when you feel that power has reached its summit, come back to the here and now and become alert and awake and refreshed."

Take the time to focus your healing resources towards the purpose of the session: enabling the client to become a non-smoker. Remember that whenever communication takes place between two individuals, most of it is conveyed and picked up unconsciously. Therefore you need to be in a positive state of belief and certainty in the client's success. The client will absorb this at an unconscious level, enhancing the prospects for the therapy.

Feel free to write your own self-hypnosis routine for preparing yourself for the client, or adapt the one above.

Ensuring a smooth session

Communication always takes place in a context, so the greater your control over all the elements of the session – both the content of the therapy and the context in which it occurs – the more effective the session is likely to be. From before the session through to their departure, do what you can to help maintain the client's calm, optimistic and confident state.

First impressions are vitally important, and influence the entire relationship you have with another person. There was an experiment where they showed a group of salespeople some video footage of a new group of colleagues whom they had not met before but with whom they would soon be working. They were then asked for their first impressions of the new staff, and whether they would enjoy working with them or not. Then these new employees joined the company and worked there for six months. At the end of the first six months, those salespeople who had watched the video footage were asked what they thought of these co-workers with whom they had been working side-by-side for six months. Amazing at it may seem, the opinions they expressed were virtually identical to the answers they had given six months previously when they had merely watched those people on video.[1]

What first impression does your client get of you? Make sure your body language shows your professionalism. Stand upright and imagine a book balanced on the top of your head. Breathe slowly and deeply from the diaphragm. Establish eye contact with your client and shake their hand reasonably firmly – there is no need for a bone-crusher or a wet fish handshake.

Almost all your clients will judge you instantly on your appearance, and like it or not (I certainly don't), this will have more impact on their state than any hypnotic techniques you use in the session. The first thing some people look at when they are introduced to a new person is that person's shoes. Make sure that yours are polished in case your client does that.

When people are expected to pay for something, they will be more willing to part with their money if the person they are paying is smartly dressed. Therefore I recommend that whenever you are doing therapy, men should wear a suit and tie; women should dress smartly but not ostentatiously, without too much jewellery. Even the colour of a suit conveys a certain psychological code in terms of the affect on the person seeing it. The darker the suit, the greater the perceived authority of the individual wearing it. The ideal colours for the hypnotherapist to wear for a smoking cessation session are mid-to-dark blue or mid-to-dark grey. Anything lighter tends to err too far on the side of informality, while black tends to come across as so authoritarian that rapport is adversely affected.

When people engage the services of members of most occupations, they generally have a preconception of what those services will cost. They expect the fees charged by a barrister for legal representation to be much higher than those charged by a gardener to maintain a garden. However, most potential clients have little preconception as to whether hypnotherapy is "supposed to be" a high-cost or a low-cost service. Therefore, the hypnotherapist can shape those expectations. The appearance of high status justifies higher prices and makes people more willing to pay those prices, thus giving the therapist a higher income. It also raises positive expectations, and, as you know, expectations tend to be realised. However, these points are valid only in a context in which the hypnotherapy is effective in achieving the client's goal. You must know your stuff and – just as important – how to apply it in response to your client's communications. But once you have mastered effective hypnotherapy, these presentational touches ensure that you exercise the maximum degree of influence for a positive outcome.

Make it easy for the client to remain in as positive a state as possible. My practice is based in a large building which has many therapy rooms over five floors, which can be difficult for visitors to navigate. Several of the practitioners in the building ask the receptionist to "send the client up" from the waiting room at the appointed time. However, some clients experience great difficulty finding the correct room. They wander through the building like lost souls, asking passers-by for directions. You are doing yourself no favours by putting your clients into such a confused and unresourceful state immediately before the session. When the receptionist informs me that my client has arrived, I personally walk in to the waiting room and call out, "Mr Smith", "Ms Jones" or whatever the client's name is. (Using "Mr" or "Ms" may seem unnecessarily formal these days. However, I still recommend that you use that style until you know the client personally. Even after that, if the client is older than you, I suggest you ask permission before using the client's first name.) When the client responds, I go up to them, shake their hand and say, "My name's David." I then escort the client to my room. If they have heavy bags, I offer to carry them; I help them remove their coat and hang it up; I offer to fetch the client a glass of water. The hypnotherapist's role is equivalent to that of a waiter in a good restaurant or hotel. Certainly the waiter may know more about the food and wine on offer, but nevertheless he is fully aware of who is paying for the whole event.

On the way to the room, I make conversation by asking, "Did you find the place all right?" and "Have you come far today?" The purpose of asking these simple, everyday questions is partly to influence the client's state by displacing any worries they may have, and partly to avoid an awkward silence. Making small talk gives you the opportunity to come across as an approachable, down-to-earth person, without appearing overly intrusive. Such conversations help build rapport by finding something you have in common with the client. You may also obtain useful information which can be utilised in the session.

For example, if in response to the question "Did you find the place all right?" the client says, "Oh, yes, my son's nursery is just round the corner from here," then I have just learned that the client has a young son of pre-school age. In the session, then, I can talk about how the client has successfully adapted to parenthood, and can therefore adapt to the non-smoking life just as easily. I will emphasise the benefit of knowing that the client is setting an excellent example to the child by becoming a non-smoker. In response to the question "Have you come far today?" the client might say, "Just a couple of miles from here. It was easy enough to cycle through the traffic." In this case, I have just learned that the client rides a bicycle. During the session, I can talk about how they mastered the art of cycling until it became unconscious knowledge, and in the same way can master the art of living as a non-smoker. It becomes possible to induce trance by talking about the most enjoyable cycle ride the client ever experienced, and to deepen that trance by describing cycling down a steep hill into a deep valley. It is far preferable to elicit information in this indirect way than by asking direct questions. Make the most of your first contact with the client to build rapport and indirectly elicit information which can be used later in the session.

If you dress in a conventional way, use these moments to make a special effort to build rapport with clients of unconventional appearance. One of my smoking-cessation clients at Harley Street was a young punk rocker with a spiky pink haircut of stegosaurus proportions, and an array of safety pins in his nose, ears and jacket. As soon as I welcomed him, I engaged in recollections of the punk rock era of the late 1970s, when I was in my teens, the controversy which surrounded bands like the Sex Pistols, and my memories of visiting the shops on the King's Road and Carnaby Street which sold punk regalia. I continued, "There again, I've kind of lost track of the punk scene since then. What's been happening recently?" This was the client's cue to talk about the concert halls and clubs he frequented, and the bands he followed. This built rapport, kept the client in his comfort zone and gave me material which I used to induce trance and access resources during the session.

Your room must be comfortable, quiet, tidy and spotlessly clean. Make sure that everything is ready before the client arrives, so that the session starts bang on time and proceeds smoothly and without interruptions. The temperature should be comfortable, and everything from business cards to forms to pens to water in place before the session begins. You lose credibility if you have to ask the client to wait while you run round tidying up or looking for a functioning pen or a box of tissues.

Home visits

The question of visiting clients in their own homes is likely to arise at some point. A few hypnotherapists only do home visits and do not practise from their own premises. Others display the phrase "home visits available" on their leaflets, advertisements, business cards and website. My preference is not to actually announce that home visits are available, but to be happy to provide them when people specifically request them.

If you provide home visits, explain that hypnotherapy is available to those who are house-bound for health reasons. Also, it saves you the cost of seeing a client at a clinic, particularly if you pay the clinic by the hour. It is also much more likely that the client will show up!

However, heavy traffic, navigation problems, parking restrictions, difficulty in finding a parking space, and the risk of crime in some areas, are all disadvantages. Set out early, and allow at least half an hour more than the time you expect it will take. It is *essential* to turn up on time – neither early nor late.

The environment in the client's home could be a drawback. The client might be distracted by children running around, music or television playing, and the telephone ringing. It is likely that there are undesirable anchors – in the NLP sense – associated with the smoking habit in the client's home. In NLP, anchoring is defined as "The process of associating an internal response with some external trigger (similar to classical conditioning) so that the response may be quickly, and sometimes covertly, reaccessed."

(By contrast, when a client visits you, you control the environment, you create positive anchors, and the very fact that the client makes a journey to visit you – outside of the client's usual daily routine – adds a degree of significance to the session for them.)

Also, when doing a home visit, you are in the slightly awkward position of "telling the person what to do" in their own home. Because the client is at home – a concept associated with continuity and security – it might be more difficult to make such a dramatic transformation as becoming a non-smoker. It is probably not decisive in itself, but an accumulation of these tiny details can make the difference between becoming a non-smoker or not.

During a home visit, do not accept the client's offer of a cup of tea or coffee. It is not for the client to be running round after you. Build rapport by saying positive things about the client's house, garden and decorations. Get on with the therapy as quickly as possible, and leave as soon as possible after receiving payment.

Chapter 5

Starting the main smoking cessation session

Listening and reframing

Hypnotherapy is no more – and also no less – than effective communication. The hypnotherapist communicates effectively by pacing and leading the client in order to get them to re-create their world in a way which better meets their needs and desires. In this sense hypnotherapy is much like the arts, cinema being a good example. A film is a re-creation of the world, which may capture the viewer's imagination if they can imagine themselves in the story. If not, it appears unconvincing and boring.

The film director Alfred Hitchcock said, "Cinema is life with the boring bits missed out." The producer Sam Goldwyn gave the following formula for a successful film: "You start with an earthquake and build up to a climax." In the same way, hypnosis is essentially communication which is optimised for maximum effectiveness at each stage, as well as being a more emotionally participatory experience for the client. The "boring bits" – the bits which do not connect with their current experience – are missed out. Also, effective hypnotherapy "starts with an earthquake" in the sense that at the very start of the session you want to jolt your client out of the engrained pattern of thought in which the problem behaviour is embedded. The hypnotherapist must have certainty – absolute, unshakable certainty – that the client is becoming a non-smoker as a result of the session, and must convey that certainty in every possible way. You must be like Queen Victoria during the Boer War when one of her advisers mentioned the possibilities of defeat. She replied, "We are not interested in the possibilities of defeat. They do not exist." That is the conviction you must take with you to every hypnotherapy session – and must convey to your client so that it comes true.

One-word reframing

Using language artfully means that you have the capacity to change the meaning of an experience simply by labelling it differently. "One-word reframing" is about changing the client's experience with a single word.

For example, a client might feel trepidation at the prospect of life without ciga-rettes. If such a client tells you that they have such concerns, then you ask the question, "How are you feeling now?" The client is likely to say "nervous" or "anxious". Your reply is, "Another word for nervous/anxious is excited." That is a one-word reframe. It re-interprets the client's experience. A person who is feeling nervous or anxious and a person who is feeling excited are going through exactly the same physiological experiences. The breathing is rapid, shallow, irregular and from the upper chest. There is tension in the muscles, particularly in the face, neck, shoulders and upper chest. The heart is beating rapidly. There may be perspiration on the palms, and such sensations as "but-terflies in the stomach" or a "knot in the stomach". Those physiological features are present in both cases. By reframing those experiences – re-labelling them with the word "excited" – you instantly change the meaning of the client's physiological experience to one that implies positive expectation.

Another example of a one-word reframe is changing the client's use of the word "addiction" to the word "habit". Avoid using the word "addiction", which tends to imply something that the client cannot get control over. If a client uses the words "addiction" or "addicted", then ask, "How would you define that word?" Typically the client might answer, "It's something that's happening outside of my control." Then you might reply, "Can you repeat what you just said, saying the word 'habit' instead of 'addiction'?" The client substitutes the suggested word. You say, "And how does that feel now?" The client is likely to say that it makes the prospect of becoming a non-smoker somewhat easier. Of course, the precise use of the words depends on what the client actually says and how.

Reframing smoking and the desire to quit in positive terms

At the start of the session, seat the client behind the desk, on which lies a form, together with at least two pens (to ensure that at least one pen works). The very act of seating the client behind the desk – where a doctor, therapist or other expert usually sits – shows the client that *they* are the expert in charge of the process of becoming a non-smoker, rather than the hypnotherapist. This insight on the client's part that the expertise rests entirely within them is the first tremor of the earthquake which begins the session. The full earthquake takes place when the client sees the form, which reads as follows:

[your name]
Clinical Hypnotherapist
[your address]
[your phone number]
[your e-mail]

Name of non-smoker _____

Address _____

The benefits I have gained from stopping smoking:

    1. _____

    2. _____

    3. _____

The money I save from being a non-smoker:

    £ _____ per week

    £ _____ per month

    £ _____ per year

I am now a non-smoker.

Signed _____

Date _____

It can indeed be quite an earthquake for many clients to describe themselves as non-smokers by filling in this form. Several of my clients over the years have assumed that it did not apply to them, and put in somebody else's name instead! Some clients say, "Well, I'm not a non-smoker yet, so how can I fill this in?" You reply, "The purpose of this is to get you to *think* of yourself as being a non-smoker." Of course, that is indeed the purpose. Through the act of actually writing down their name next to "name of non-smoker," the client becomes an active participant in the process of becoming a non-smoker. It tends to undermine or eliminate the scepticism, cynicism and detachment which many clients bring to the session. In writing that they are a non-smoker, the client becomes an active collaborator in the therapeutic process. The client is there because they hope to become a non-smoker. By getting the client to fill in the form, you are strengthening that part that believes in the possibility of becoming a non-smoker by obtaining that written assumption and commitment. The process of filling in the form draws the client in to greater involvement with the session. Also, information which is written down is stored in a different part of the brain from information which is heard – so the client is having the knowledge that they are a non-smoker encoded in two places.

Do not ask for any more information than the client's name and address. Your client's privacy is of paramount importance. When dealing with the specific issue of smoking cessation, do not ask for the client's age, occupation, marital status, name of GP or any other information.

Below the address is "The benefits I have gained from stopping smoking". Here there are two purposes: first, to shift the client's attention during the session towards the desired outcome, and, second, to identify the values which are specifically most important to this particular client in achieving that outcome.

The focus of the session from this point on is to achieve the goals which the client has written down. As each client is unique, it is likely that there will be a wide variety in the goals desired by different clients, although "health" and "saving money" come up most often. As well as orienting the client's thinking towards these positive goals, you will also feed back to them later what they have written down, when you induce trance.

Then the client is asked to add up "The money I save from being a non-smoker" by week, month and year. Many people have difficulty in carrying out even quite simple arithmetic. However, do not provide them with a calculator, because you want them to go through the effort of actually mentally calculating the total amount they will be saving as non-smokers. If somebody says, "My maths is terrible," then simply reply, "Oh, that's all right. It's not an exam – it won't be marked. The purpose is just to show people how much they're saving now they're becoming non-smokers." Obviously, here you are making a pre-supposition that the client will become a non-smoker. Also, you use the third person – "people" rather than "you". Avoid using the word "you" too often in hypnotherapy. Many people might find it a bit direct and intrusive, and it can sometimes lead to scepticism. If the client repeatedly hears the word "you", then they are likely to start thinking, "How can this therapist claim to know these things about me? He/she doesn't know anything about me." However, if you use words like "people", "we", "a non-smoker", "a person who used to smoke", then clients automatically relate what you are saying to themselves uncritically. Everyone tends to relate what they hear to themselves, even when it is superficially about "people" in general or a specific other person. It is as if there is a filter in everyone's minds asking, "How does this relate or compare to me and my situation?"

So use the third person if you want to get a point across subtly but effectively. When you say, "The point of that [calculation of savings] is to show how much people will save when they become non-smokers," the client interprets that as meaning, "The point of that is to show *me* how much *I* will save now that *I'm* becoming a non-smoker." In other words, the client internalises the presupposition that they are becoming a non-smoker.

Note that you are focusing on the positive benefits of becoming, and living as, a non-smoker. There is no mention at any point in the session of the health problems caused by the smoking habit.

Then ask your client to take a seat in one of the two armchairs which are facing each other. Have the chairs in the "social zone" of 1.2 to 3.6 metres apart, which, according to Edward Hall, is best for formal and impersonal interactions.[1] This places you at the right distance to see the client's entire seated body at the same time. You do not want to have to keep scanning them, which would happen if they were too close, nor miss the details if you were too far away. As you glance down the form, you say, "Good, excellent" – regardless of what they have written. Simply saying these positive words helps to validate the client and give them a positive feeling. Obviously, the client assumes that you are expressing approval of what they have written. Then you put the form to one side, but keep it within easy reach for use later, and start to speak to the client.

If the client is older than you, ask, "Do you mind if I call you by your first name?" Even in this day and age, it is courteous to do so. It enables the client to give permission for the relative informality of being on first-name terms. If the client is about the same age as, or noticeably younger than you are, then it is fine to use first-name terms without asking permission. Often I will read the name on the form and if it's Jeffrey or Susan, I ask, "Shall I call you Jeffrey/ Susan?" The client will then often say, "It's usually Jeff/Sue" – so you use the nickname. With an unusual name like Siobhan, you might want to ask for the correct pronunciation, and make sure you repeat it correctly.

Build rapport by being respectful and using the name they want to be called by. Avoid being too familiar; do not intrude upon their privacy.

The session itself

The exact course of a smoking cessation session cannot be predicted in advance. Nevertheless, there are certain key ideas and techniques which it is important to get across to most clients during the session. Your task is to ensure that by the end of the session, the client has become a non-smoker through unconscious learning and also that they have learned techniques which enable them to control and change subjective experiences so as to stay a non-smoker in every conceivable situation.

Most clients expect the therapist to take the initiative by asking questions. The following is a broad outline of how to guide the session when this situation takes place. It needs to be adapted somewhat for each client, depending on their individual experiences and needs.

Some clients, as soon as they sit down, will initiate the conversation. They spontaneously start talking about their present experience of smoking, their previous attempts to quit the habit, or their concerns about how to deal with issues such as stress, over-eating or socialising with smokers once they become non-smokers. If so, talk about the subject which the client mentions, but gently guide the direction of the session so that you still get the essential message and techniques across, albeit in a different order from that presented below.

If you are initiating the conversation, ask, "Can you tell me how you first started smoking?" The client then gives you a description of how they started. In most cases, it was as a teenager; in a minority of cases, it was as a young adult. Whatever the client's experience, validate and reframe it. If the person started as a teenager, you could say the following, providing that it is congruent with the description the client has just provided:

> "Every problem was once a solution. When people start smoking, it does something positive for them. Eighty-two percent of people who smoke today started in their teenage years. At that time in life, young people want to prove themselves, be part of the gang, rebel against authority, seem to be more grown-up than they really are. Smoking comes across as being cool, glamorous and sophisticated."

If the person started as an adult, then depending on the client's account, you could say,

> "Every problem was once a solution. When you started smoking, it did something positive for you. Eighteen percent of people who smoke today started as adults. It can often be to form a bond with a group of friends who smoke, or in a workplace where there's a strong sense of camaraderie, like the armed forces, or the police or fire service, even a hospital."

Then continue:

> "These are all positive intentions. Your unconscious mind accepted smoking as the best, the most immediately available way, of achieving those positive intentions. At that time, it worked. What we're going to do today is to find a new, more useful way of achieving those positive intentions than the habit of smoking. When we talk about the unconscious mind, we mean everything that you're

not aware of now. The *conscious* mind has only limited awareness at any given moment. Everything else is unconscious. It includes your memories, your beliefs, your habits, your values, your imagination, your representations of the future. It includes everything happening in your body that you don't need to consciously think about: your heartbeat, pulse, the circulation of blood, the digestion of food, the immune system – thousands of functions all going on outside of conscious awareness, but all coordinated. The unconscious is where real learning takes place." (Short pause.) "Can you remember the first cigarette you ever had?"

Some clients say, "No". In that case you say,

"Well, typically, when people start smoking, they cough, they feel sick, their eyes water, they often turn green. That's because the body's defence mechanisms were trying to defend you against that poison. But pretty soon, the body adapts to the habit of smoking and comes to expect all those cigarettes coming in."

Others say, "Yes". If they do, you ask, "What was that like?" Most clients say that it tasted unpleasant, that they felt dizzy and sick, but a minority will say that they took to it instantly and maybe positively enjoyed it. In the latter case – assuming their recollections are correct – it means that the client was in such a state of hypnotic rapture about the joy of becoming a smoker – and obtaining the positive benefits which the unconscious mind associated with smoking – that the body's physical defence mechanisms were simply overridden. In that event you can either give the above explanation or just say, "Right," and go on to the next section.

If the client says, "Yes" and recalls a bad experience, then you say,

"Your body was doing its best to defend you. Typically, when people start smoking, they cough, they feel sick, their eyes water, they often turn green – that's because the body's defence mechanisms are trying to defend them against that poison. But pretty soon, the body adapts to the habit of smoking and comes to expect all those cigarettes coming in."

Whatever the person recalls about the first cigarette (if anything), continue:

"There's a thing called the nicotine trick. It happens by chance that the chemical effect of nicotine on the body is very similar to that of fear or anxiety. When a person smokes their first cigarette, it takes about four hours for the effect to kick in. The person feels a tightness in the muscles, especially around the face, the neck, the shoulders and the upper chest. The heart beats more quickly, and there may be perspiration on the palms. There is a knot in the stomach, and a general sense of unease. This is actually the chemical effect of the nicotine on the body, but it seems like fear or anxiety. So a lot of young people after their first cigarette say, 'Hey, I don't like this, I'm not smoking any more of those.' So they let the nicotine leave the body and pretty soon they're back to normal. But other young people feel that same feeling and think, 'I don't like this feeling – I'm going to have another cigarette to calm me down.' So they have a second cigarette and all that does is re-set the process, so that they go back to the start and it takes another four hours for that nicotine effect to set in. And then when they feel that sensation that seems like fear or anxiety again, they reach for a third cigarette, and so on – until the day that they stop. And when they stop, the body gets a breathing space where the nicotine leaves the system and the body returns to the state it was in before the person ever smoked that first cigarette."

This is all true. The purpose of saying this is to help your client understand precisely that the whole smoking habit – at least in its physiological aspects – rests on a trick – the simple fact that the effect of nicotine on the body seems like the experience of fear or anxiety. Because you are also talking about stopping smoking and giving the body a breathing space, the client relates that to their own situation as their imagination increasingly opens up to the idea of becoming a non-smoker. Note that throughout the session you are talking exclusively in terms of success, and in terms of how people become non-smokers, as if it is the easiest and most natural thing in the world, and presupposing success in the case of the client.

Utilising previous success in quitting

Hypnotherapy is about seeking and utilising the client's resources. If the client has previously stopped smoking for more than two weeks, then the memory of that experience is about the single most powerful resource that will enable them to become a non-smoker.

You continue: "Have you stopped smoking for any length of time since you started?" What you are looking for is any experience in which the client has stopped smoking for a period of at least two weeks. It takes two weeks for the body to eliminate all the accumulated tar, nicotine and carbon monoxide and to become a non-smoker's body. For the client, that is a reality – it does not have to be imagined. In hypnotherapy, the memory of an actual experience is always more powerful than an imaginary experience. We remember not merely in our minds, but also in our muscles and organs.

If the client says that they stopped smoking for some length of time in the past, then ask, "How did you do that?" The client then gives you a description. It could be from the withdrawal-oriented therapy (WOT) favoured by the National Health Service, the use of nicotine replacement therapy (NRT) products (gum, lozenges, inhalers or patches), or from attending the Allen Carr seminar or reading his book *The Easy Way to Stop Smoking* (it is essential for you to read that book, by the way), or from acupuncture, or hypnotherapy or from a moment of transformation in which the person really decided, in a highly motivated state, to become a non-smoker – and it happened. Quite often it was in the context of a major event in the client's life. Such a client's description might be, "When I moved into the new house, it all seemed so new, clean and immaculate that it was like starting a new way of life. I just decided not to smoke any more, and that was as simple as that. Didn't smoke for five years after that."

It is important here to pace the client's previous success by mentioning the difference between hypnotherapy on the one hand and the client's previous method (other than hypnotherapy) which helped them stop smoking in the past. Always talk of other smoking cessation methods and therapists in positive terms. They are doing good work, and every method has indeed enabled millions of people to become non-smokers. Here is the approach to take with each of the major methods, which the client may previously have used for a time.

Withdrawal-oriented therapy (WOT)

This is provided by the NHS, and was developed by the Institute of Psychiatry. You can tell the client:

> "The basic principle of withdrawal-oriented therapy is to treat tobacco smoking as a form of drug addiction. It focuses on helping you through the withdrawal symptoms experienced during the two weeks immediately following quitting. Often they give you medication to deal with those cravings and group sessions to give mutual support. Undoubtedly, it has helped many people stop smoking. But it doesn't deal with unconscious part of the mind, or enable you to ensure that you stay a non-smoker in all situations. With hypnotherapy, we're dealing with the unconscious part of the mind, so that your body understands that you are a non-smoker and welcomes the opportunity to expel all the poisons which have been trapped inside. Also, we'll be doing self-hypnosis, which is a way of creating a calm, relaxed, resourceful state any time you want it, so that you will stay a non-smoker in all situations."

Nicotine-replacement therapies (NRT)

This is generally favoured by officialdom and often used as part of WOT. You can tell the client:

> "A lot of people have undoubtedly been helped to become non-smokers by using nicotine patches/inhalers/gums/lozenges [whatever method the client used]. The way they work is suppressing the cravings by putting nicotine into

the system in smaller and smaller doses. And of course they only deal with the physical aspects of the problem, not with the unconscious mind. What we want to do is get the nicotine out of the system and deal with the psychological aspect of the habit, so that you learn to live as a non-smoker at an unconscious level. Also, we'll be doing self-hypnosis, which is a way of creating a calm, relaxed, resourceful state any time you want it, so that you will stay a non-smoker in all situations."

Reading Allen Carr's **The Easy Way to Stop Smoking**

You can tell the client:

"Yes, over seven million copies of that book have been sold, and many have stopped smoking immediately as a result of reading it. When you read that book, the unconscious part of your mind learned about the reality of smoking and carried out an internal process of transformation which made you a non-smoker instantly. Yet that book is merely ink on paper. You see how your unconscious mind can make such a massive transformation based purely on an idea expressed in words on a page? We're going to tap into that same ability of your unconscious mind to repeat the success you previously enjoyed and to make sure that you're well protected in order to stay a non-smoker in all future situations."

Attending an Allen Carr group seminar

You can tell the client:

"The Allen Carr seminars can be very useful because you get group dynamics, a sense of camaraderie, and the support of other members of the group. The message is much the same as the book, and you get twenty minutes of hypnotherapy at the end. But the advantage of the individual therapy which we're doing today is that it is tailored to you as a unique individual. We want to repeat the success you enjoyed at that seminar and ensure that you have techniques immediately available in every future situation in order to remain a non-smoker."

Acupuncture

This is still relatively uncommon as a smoking cessation method, but you will get a few who have had acupuncture. You can ask the client:

"Did they put a small metal object in your ear?" (Acupuncturists use a variety of objects, including needles, to apply pressure to different points on the body.

Avoid saying the word "needles", because some clients might dislike the idea of needles penetrating the body.) "They probably explained that the purpose of that is to redirect the *chi* energy along the meridians of the body. These concepts from traditional Chinese medicine seem to correspond very closely to the electrical currents flowing through the body. What we're going to do today is ask your unconscious mind to remember how you stopped smoking that time and to repeat that process. We also want to make sure that you also have techniques immediately available in every future situation so that you stay a non-smoker for life."

Hypnotherapy

You can tell the client:

"The great thing is that you've proved that you can become a non-smoker through unconscious communication. When you went to see that hypnotherapist, your unconscious mind carried out an internal transformation which made you a non-smoker easily. What we're going to do is repeat that success. But this time, I'd like to show you how you can use self-hypnosis so that you'll be able to put yourself into that relaxed, resourceful, comfortable state any time you want and *stay* a non-smoker in all future situations."

A spontaneous moment of internal change

You can tell the client:

"Congratulations. As we go through life, we all experience these key moments where a transformation takes place and it all just comes together. Just like learning to walk or run or swim or read or drive a car. There can be moments of high motivation in which everything simply comes together at an unconscious level and it happens instantly and easily. What we want to do today is to bring back that moment, repeat your success and this time ensure that you have – instantly available to you – the ability to remain a non-smoker for good."

Whatever description of how they previously stopped the client gives, you say,

"Well, the great thing is that you have actually done it. You gave your body that breathing space, it got rid of all that poison, and you actually lived as a non-smoker for that length of time. Your unconscious mind and your body have powerful memories of that experience. What we're going to do today is ask the unconscious mind to repeat that transformation, but this time make sure that it's a permanent one. Can you remember what life was like during those three weeks/six months/two years when you were a non-smoker? How did you feel?"

The client will probably give you a description of their memories of life as a non-smoker. In most cases, people will tell you that they felt physically fitter, that their breathing was much easier, and that they enjoyed a greater sense of freedom. Take a careful mental note of the words and phrases the client uses, because you are going to feed them back later in the session. The client might recall a specific experience such as being able to go jogging without getting out of breath, or looking in the mirror and enjoying the sight of clean, white teeth, or just feeling a general internal sense of achievement.

If the client does have good memories of life as an ex-smoker for that length of time, then you say,

> "Excellent. Those experiences are very much part of your life. We don't just store memories in our head – they're also in the muscles, in the organs, in every part of the body. What we're going to do in a few moments is to ask the unconscious mind to repeat that transformation, but this time to make sure that you're well protected so that you stay a non-smoker in all future situations."

In a minority of cases, the client will tell you that they cannot remember, or did not notice, any difference. In that case you say,

> "Well, the memory of life as a non-smoker is there at an unconscious level. It's reality, it's a part of your life. What we're going to do in a few moments is to ask the unconscious mind to repeat that transformation, but this time to make sure that you're well protected, so that you stay a non-smoker in all future situations."

Again, you are validating the client, building positive expectations and the (well-founded) belief that they will indeed successfully become a non-smoker and stay one.

Then you ask, "What happened at the end of those three months/two years/ etc, that led you to go back to smoking?" The client might tell you that they experienced a stressful or difficult situation, or went out drinking with friends and assumed it was possible to have "just the one" cigarette, or else met an old friend who was still smoking and accepted a cigarette "for old time's sake". Whatever the situation was that led to the return to smoking, validate it:

> "Well, the great thing is that you have proved that you can do it, that you can live as a non-smoker. What we want to do today is to repeat that success, but this time make sure that you're well prepared to stay a non-smoker in all future situations."

If the client has never stopped smoking since the day they started, then you still validate them in the same way. You say,

> "The great thing is that you did live as a non-smoker for the first fifteen years [or whatever age the client started] of your life. Your body, your unconscious mind, have got powerful memories of what it was like living as a young child, as a young teenager, year after year, growing, learning, playing, socialising, travelling, in which you never once even thought about smoking or cigarettes. What we are going to do in a few moments is ask the unconscious part of your mind to bring back that healthy way of living, but this time make sure that you're well protected, so that you stay a non-smoker in all future situations."

In both cases – whether the client has previously stopped smoking or not – validate their experience and utilise it. Place the power to live as a non-smoker firmly where it belongs – with the client himself or herself.

A fundamental rule of hypnotherapy is this: a real experience which is remembered is always more powerful than an imagined experience.

Eliciting strategies (from NLP)

Then move on to the next step, which is asking the client about their recent smoking habit. You say, "If we talk about recently, the last few weeks or so, how many cigarettes have you been smoking on a typical day?" The client might say, "Five", "Ten", or "Twenty." Whatever number the client gives, you say,

> "The great news is that we only have to focus on the first cigarette of the day. Once you're free from the desire for that first cigarette, the other [four, nine, nineteen, etc] don't even come into the picture. Have you had a cigarette this morning?"

If the client says, "Yes", then continue, "What time was the first cigarette you had today?" Whatever time the client gives, you reply, "Can you tell me what went through your mind at eight o'clock/nine-thirty this morning when you reached for that cigarette?"

What we are seeking here is a strategy (in NLP terms) which shows how the client experiences the process of desiring, reaching for and lighting a cigarette. In NLP, a strategy is defined as "a set of explicit mental and behavioural steps used to achieve a specific outcome." The most important aspect of a strategy is the *representational systems* used to carry out the specific steps. If you have studied NLP you will know that strategy elicitation can be quite complicated. It is a question of analysing, breaking down into a sequence, the thoughts in a person's mind which lead them either to do something beneficial, such as

achieving good results in sports or business or music – or something less beneficial, such as smoking a cigarette. If possible, you are going to show the client
how to get control of that process and turn it to their benefit. If the client can
identify the stimulus or trigger that gets them to reach for a cigarette, then that
is something you can work with. In that case, move on to the section below
relating to changing submodalities. If the client seems to be struggling to identify such an internal trigger, then prompt them by saying,

> "Every time we have a habit, whether it's a useful habit or a less useful one,
> there's a signal inside which triggers it off. Some people hear a little voice in
> their head saying, 'It's eight o'clock in the morning, time for a cigarette.' Some
> people experience a tightness in the throat or an empty feeling in the stomach.
> Others see a lighted cigarette in their mind's eye. Is there anything like that that
> you are aware of?"

If the client says "Yes" and gives you a description, then move on to the section
on changing submodalities. If the client says "No, it's just a habit/automatic,
etc", then validate that by saying, "Yes, it's become unconscious." Then ignore
the submodality work and simply move on to the next section.

When you ask the question, "Can you tell me what went through your mind
at eight o'clock/nine-thirty this morning when you reached for that cigarette?"
a significant proportion of clients will say something like, "Well, I knew I was
coming to see you today, so I thought, 'This is the last morning that I'm ever
going to be doing this.'" If the client says something like that, then just say,
"Excellent", and move on to the next section, ignoring submodalities.

But in the event that the client can and does get in touch with the internal trigger which leads to them reaching for a cigarette, then you have an exceptionally
powerful technique for bringing about their transformation towards being a
non-smoker. In practice, you may find that only about half of your clients are
able to notice and change the submodalities of their internal strategies.

Changing submodalities

Changing submodalities is one of the techniques that came out of the early
years of NLP. In practice, a majority of your clients will not be used to examining their internal experiences, and may find it difficult to analyse their internal
strategies and change their submodalities in the context of one session with
you. Do not try and force this. Apply the "three second rule". With any technique you use in therapy, give it three seconds to connect with the client. If at
the end of three seconds, the client is simply not connecting with or understanding the technique, or is "lost", simply validate them by saying, "That's
fine," and move immediately on to a different technique. If you try and persist

with a technique which the client is simply not getting for more than three seconds, you are damaging rapport and the client is losing confidence in you. Move on to a technique that the client can connect with.

However, with those clients who can work with internal strategies and sub-modalities, you have a very powerful way in which they can take a major step forward towards becoming and remaining non-smokers.

Every habit requires a particular event or experience to trigger it. Once we recognise that trigger, we can change its nature by consciously adjusting its sub-modalities. This altered trigger will have a different effect on us. In the case of a person who smokes, let's say that they identify a voice in the head which says, "It's eight o'clock in the morning, time for a cigarette." You ask, "Can you hear that voice now?" If the client says, "No", then you ask, "Can you *remember* that voice now?" If the client says, "Yes", and they can remember it, then continue working with submodalities. (If the client says, "No", then skip the submodalities.) Then ask, "Whose voice is it?"

The client might say, "Mine."

"And where exactly is that voice?"

The client might point to the left side of their head and say, "Here."

Reply, "On the left hand side of your head."

Then start adjusting the submodalities.

"Can you slow that voice down, so that it's like a CD being played at the wrong speed?" Slow your own voice to show what you mean. Give the client all the time that that takes, then move on.

"Can you turn the volume down, as if you were turning down the volume on a CD player, so that you can hardly hear it?"

Once the client has done that, continue: "Can you move that voice from the left hand side of your head to the right hand side?"

Once the client affirms that they have done that, you continue: "Now can you focus on that spot on the left hand side of your head where that voice was?"

Once the client affirms, you say,

> "And can you put a new voice in that same position, your own voice. Can you get that voice to say, 'It's great to be a healthy, happy non-smoker. It's great to

be a healthy, happy non-smoker.' Can you have your own voice say that in a confident, reassuring tone of voice? Can you put that voice in stereo, so that it's on both the left and right hand sides of your head? And I wonder if there's a piece of music that you find inspiring, that you can play in the background as an accompaniment as you hear that voice again and again. (Pause.) And what affect does it have on you now?"

As the client makes these submodality changes, you will probably be able to see their facial expression change, and they may start to smile or even laugh. They may say something like, "I feel much calmer" or, "It feels good." Then you say, "You see how easy it is to get control over our internal impulses and get them to work for our benefit?" Note that you are communicating to the client in the form of questions. For example, "Can you move it from the left hand side of your head to the right hand side?"

There are three reasons for this. First, it maintains rapport. If it turns out that the client cannot make the change you are requesting, they will simply say, "No", so you say, "That's okay", and rapport is maintained. Second, it encourages a response. If someone asks you a question, automatically your mind gets active in seeking an answer – which is not necessarily the case if you simply make a factual statement or give an instruction. Third, it avoids giving the impression that you are giving the client orders – as if you were a doctor or a sergeant-major. A lay hypnotherapist is by definition not a doctor, and even if it happens that you *were* a sergeant-major in the army, it is still best to use this question-based approach when dealing with hypnotherapy clients who are paying for your services. (If you do have experience as a sergeant-major, this will come in very handy when you need to adopt a more authoritarian approach later in the session!)

The example above deals with changing *auditory* submodalities. The only auditory submodalities we need to be concerned with are position, volume, speed, tone of voice, and of course content – the actual words the voice says. The voice does have other qualities, but adding more is likely to confuse your client. Concern yourself with position, volume, speed, tone of voice and words only. The words, "And I wonder if there's a piece of music that you find inspiring, that you can play in the background as an accompaniment as you hear that voice again and again" are a question in the form of a statement. If the client does have a piece of music which they find inspiring, then if they can "play" that music in the imagination while listening to the affirmation, "It's great to be a healthy, happy non-smoker", then this will strengthen the impact of that affirmation. If the client does not come up with such a piece of music, then the fact that you have phrased it as "I wonder …" implies that it's not particularly important one way or the other, and therefore no big deal if there is no music.

The same principles apply in the event that the client's strategy involves kinesthetic submodalities. For example, the client might identify their internal trigger to reach for a cigarette as being a feeling in the stomach. In that case, you ask, "Are you aware of that feeling now?" If the client says "Yes", then continue. If the reply is "No", then ask, "Can you remember that feeling now?" If "No", then skip submodalities.

If "Yes", then you ask,

> "What size is that feeling?"

The client might reply,

> "It's about the size of a tennis ball."

> "Is it heavy or light?"

> "Heavy."

> "What temperature is it?"

> "Cold."

> "Does it have a colour?"

> "Yes, it's black."

> "Is there any movement in it?"

> "Yes, it moves up from the base of the stomach to the throat."

Then you reply,

> "Excellent. Can you shrink that feeling down, so that it's very small, the size of a pea?"

Let the client do that.

> "Can you reduce its weight, making it lighter and lighter?"

> "Can you paint it a light, bright colour?"

Let the client do that. (Obviously a pea is light in weight and green in colour, so you have more or less suggested those new submodalities.)

"Can you warm it up, as if a hot fire is underneath it?"

Let the client do that.

"Can you reverse its movement, so that it moves from the throat down to the base of the stomach?"

Let the client do that.

"And what effect does it have on you now?"

"Kind of strange."

"Does it make you want to have a cigarette?"

"No."

"You see how easy it is to change our internal experiences? Just by doing exactly what you just did, you can transform that feeling so that it has a completely different affect."

Note that the only kinesthetic submodalities you need to use are position, size, weight, temperature, movement and colour: any more is likely to "throw" or "lose" your client.

In my experience, it is only occasionally that the strategic cue to smoke a cigarette is in the visual modality. On the rare occasions when the client experiences such a visual cue, of course the principle is the same. It could go like this.

The client might say,

"I see a picture of myself sitting at the breakfast table, the coffee in one hand, the cigarette in the other."

You would say,

"That picture – where is it?"

"Right ahead of me, about three feet away."

"Is it colour or black-and-white?"

"Colour."

"How large is it?"

"Pretty big."

"Is it brightly lit or dark?"

"Brightly lit."

"It is a moving picture or still?"

"Moving."

"Fine. Can you freeze-frame it, so that it becomes a still picture?"

"Yes."

"Can you put that picture in black and white?"

"Yes."

"Can you darken it, as if you're turning down the brightness knob on a television set?"

"Yes."

"Can you shrink it down, so that it's the size of a postage stamp?"

"Yes."

"Can you make that picture blurred and out of focus and somewhat scratched, like an old photo?"

"Yes."

"Can you move it so that it's ten feet away from you?"

"Yes."

"And what effect does it have on you now?"

"It doesn't bother me so much."

"Does it make you want a cigarette now?"

"No."

"Excellent. You see how easy it is to change your inner representations?"

Likewise, in the visual modality, you only need work with the picture's position, size, brightness and focus, and whether it is moving or still, colour or black-and-white and focus. Any more, and your client could find it too much to deal with.

Daily routines and ultradian rhythms

Whether the client can change the trigger through submodalities or not, you ask, "Can you tell me what sort of situations in a typical day that you've been smoking recently, let's say, the last few weeks?" The client then gives you a description of the kind of situations they have been smoking in recently. This description is likely to give you a considerable amount of information about the client's lifestyle and daily routine without you having to be so intrusive as to ask for it. You may find out whether the client works, and if so in what occupation, or whether the client looks after the children, as well as other information which should not be asked for directly.

Take a careful mental note of the client's replies. Your task at this point is partly to pace the client and get across the idea that the habit can be replaced with a more useful alternative at each point, and partly to gather information about the client's smoking habit which you will feed back later in trance.

Some clients smoke from the moment they wake up to the moment they go to sleep. Others start smoking only once they arrive at their workplace, or after lunch, or only in the evenings. Remember what the client tells you, so that the rest of the session is tailored to their actual experience. Once the client's description is over, you reassure the client by saying:

> "People often smoke in order to mark the different shifts during the day. They will say, 'This is my "getting ready in the morning" cigarette that I have with my coffee,' 'This the cigarette I have to face commuting,' 'This is my "focusing energy on arrival at work" cigarette,' 'This is my after-lunch cigarette,' 'This is my "winding down in the evening" cigarette,' 'This is my socialising cigarette,' 'This is my "getting ready for sleep" cigarette.' The fact is that nicotine is in fact a stimulant, but people smoke both in order to increase their level of energy and to create relaxation. What we want to do is to find a better, more useful way of preparing ourselves for the different situations we face day-to-day than the habit of smoking.

> "As we go through the day, we experience what's called ultradian rhythms. What this means is that we are intently focused on what we are doing for about ninety minutes, then the mind naturally wants a break, a shift in attention, a moment to oneself, for about fifteen minutes, then there's another ninety minutes of intent focus, then another fifteen minutes' break, and so on, throughout the day."

You illustrate this by "drawing" in the air a series of "hills" and "valleys" to make the point. Continue by saying:

"It's typically in those valleys in between those hills when the smoker has their cigarettes. But non-smokers have their own ways of giving themselves a break every 90 minutes. They might have tea or coffee or water, go and talk to someone, walk around a bit. What we need is a more useful way of marking those breaks than the habit of smoking." (Short pause.) "Would you say that, recently, you've smoked in order to change your mood?"

If the client says, "No", then you just say, "Fine", and skip the next section on stress management. If the client says, for instance, "Yes – I smoke when I'm stressed/bored/anxious, etc," or otherwise mentions stress or the changing of an emotion, then use the technique described in the next chapter.

Refuting the willpower myth

A number of clients will talk about willpower. They may ask you whether willpower is necessary in order to become a non-smoker, or merely assume that it is. A client might say, for example, "I just hope I've got enough willpower to make a success of it this time." If the client mentions willpower in this way, then it is essential to correct the fallacy that willpower is necessary – or even helpful – in the process of becoming a non-smoker. The way to do this is to say:

"With hypnotherapy, we really want to get away from the whole area of willpower. The problem with willpower is that it means that you're consciously focused on what you *don't* want. A person who's using willpower is constantly thinking, 'I'm definitely not going to smoke today.' 'I'm not going to accept that offer of a cigarette.' 'When I go past that shop on the corner, I'm definitely not going to go inside and buy a pack of cigarettes.' Now the unconscious part of the mind has difficulty in dealing with a negative. If you think about what you *don't* want, then you have to create a representation of it, and somehow negate that. If I say to you, 'Don't think about pink elephants,' it's obvious what goes through your mind. You have to first think of a pink elephant and then maybe cross it out, or paint it blue, or pull a curtain over it. But if I hadn't mentioned pink elephants, you probably wouldn't have thought about them all day – unless you happened to see one walking down Oxford Street" [or a nearby thoroughfare to your practice].

"The point is that we want to enable the unconscious part of your mind to carry out a process of learning which takes you forward to a future where you have simply ceased to have any interest in cigarettes. It's a bit like jelly [jello in the US]. Young children are really interested in jelly – its bright colours, its sugary taste, the way it wobbles on a plate. But the time comes when they become teenagers and adults and they simply lose interest in jelly. Probably, when you were a very young boy/girl, you were really fascinated by jelly, but I bet that if you walked through a room of young kids eating jelly, you wouldn't have to use willpower and say, 'I'm definitely not going to jump in there and eat any of that jelly.' You've simply left that interest in jelly back in the past.

"It's exactly the same with smoking. What we are going to do is ask your unconscious mind to take you forward so that that smoking habit goes back in the past where it belongs, and you move forward to a healthy, happy non-smoking future."

Living with a smoker/friends that smoke

Many clients will tell you that they live with a smoker, either a partner or people they share a home with. Others will be concerned that they regularly work or socialise with a group of smokers. Your task is to reassure the client that they will be able to successfully stay a non-smoker despite these facts.

So if the client's partner is a smoker, you can say:

"There was a survey in the States of couples who lived together for over thirty years during which one partner was a smoker and the other was a non-smoker. They found that it was quite possible for the non-smoker to live with the smoker and stay completely healthy and remain a non-smoker. Now that you're becoming a non-smoker, your body's natural defence mechanisms will come back. You can trust your body to protect you from the physical presence of any smoke in the atmosphere, and by cultivating the habit of self-hypnosis, you can ensure that you can create a calm, relaxed, resourceful state any time you want it. And remember that you only really need to deal with your own experience. Ultimately, we can never really control other people. But we *can* control our own internal experiences. Every relationship is based on finding a compromise between two distinct, unique individuals. Both partners have their own life histories, preferences, tastes and ideals, which are not going to be the same in every respect. Every successful relationship is based on awareness of the common ground and the areas where they are distinct. So of course it would be great if your partner, too, chooses to become a non-smoker at some point in the future. But what's most important for now is to recognise that you can become and stay a non-smoker no matter what your partner may or may not do in future."

Asking about smoking to change mood

When you ask clients whether they smoke a cigarette to change their mood, many will reply that they smoke when they feel stressed, or possibly they will use a word such as "nervous", "anxious" or "tense". Others will mention the issue of stress spontaneously, without you needing to ask about it. If the client does mention stress, then it is important to deal with it. In that case, proceed to the technique called rapid variable stress management, incorporated into the teaching of self-hypnosis, which is presented in the next chapter for use with such clients.

If the client specifically tells you that they *do not* smoke into order to change their mood, then it important *not* to do stress management. In that case, teach the client the simple version of instant self-hypnosis at the beginning of the following chapter.

Utilising an existing relaxation or meditation practice

If a client mentions that they already do a form of relaxation or meditation, then utilise that in inducing trance. Obviously, if a person already has a method for entering a form of trance which they have practised and enjoyed many times, it is going to be both easier for the client and more effective for the session to utilise that experience. Whether they call it "trance" or "hypnosis" is irrelevant. Quite often, when you show the client how to carry out the self-hypnosis exercise described in the next chapter, they will say something like, "It's just like doing yoga/transcendental meditation/Buddhist chanting/autogenic training," or whatever.

Match your communication to what the client says. You could say,

> "Excellent. Meditation is an Eastern technique in which essentially you clear your mind by thinking of nothing, or of a mantra, or of a lily floating on a pond, leading to a relaxed state of inner awareness in mind, body and spirit. Self-hypnosis is a Western technique in which we bring about that relaxed state of inner awareness for a reason – in order to bring about a specific improvement which you want to achieve."

Chapter 6

Educating the client to gain control

Teaching instant self-hypnosis

If the client has not mentioned the issue of stress as being something they need to deal with in connection with quitting smoking, then here is how to teach them self-hypnosis.

You say to the client:

> "Now we're going to do a simple technique called instant self-hypnosis. This is a way of putting yourself into a peaceful, calm, comfortable state any time you like. Are you comfortable in that chair?"

The client will probably say, "Yes". If not, ensure that they get comfortable. Continue:

> "Good. Now the central aspect of instant self-hypnosis is breathing in the best possible way. And we also want to ensure that the circulation of blood goes right down to the toes. So could we have both your feet on the floor, please?"

It is usually best for the client's legs to be uncrossed, with both feet on the floor. However, if you are a male therapist and your client is female, wearing a short skirt and with her legs crossed, do not ask her to put both feet on the floor.

Continue:

> "Excellent. And I want to make sure that your head is exactly aligned over your body. Now there's a point where your head feels as if it has no weight. So can you find that point where it feels as if your head is weightless and leave it there, please."

The therapist moves their own head slightly from side to side to demonstrate.

> "Good. Now your head is exactly aligned over your body, so your breathing is at its best. Now with your *eyes closed*, I'd like you to focus on your breathing. Breathe slowly, deeply and evenly, building up a nice, natural rhythm of deep, easy breathing. That's right. And the best place to breathe from is your diaphragm, which is just beneath your ribcage, as you probably already know. And

as you're breathing from the diaphragm, so your stomach is going up and down, and that's just fine, because it means that oxygen is flowing to every part of the body, which is exactly what the body needs. Good. And every time you breathe out, can you expel all the air from your lungs, breathing in completely new air, so that you're getting a really good air circulation. That's right. And every time you breathe out, in your own mind, say the word "calm" to yourself, silently and mentally. And every time you breathe out, see the word "calm", written right in front of you, written in your mind's eye. Good. And every time you do this, you'll be putting yourself into a peaceful, calm, comfortable state.

"And if you can find twenty minutes a day to practise doing this, maybe first thing in the morning, during some break in the day, perhaps when you come home in the evening, or maybe last thing at night, then you'll be training your body in the habit of relaxation, which will have excellent long-term health benefits for you.

"And as you continue to enjoy this experience of instant self-hypnosis, you can be aware that everything you experience is authentic, there's no right or wrong in any of this. And all your memories are stored away, something like photos in a pile of old albums. Colour photos and black-and-white, big blow-ups and small prints, digital photos and Polaroids, pictures stretching way back throughout the course of your life, all stored away in that pile of albums. And your unconscious mind has full access to all those images."

This photo album metaphor is used because it is something everyone can relate to. We are all familiar with the idea of putting photographs in albums as a way of keeping memories of events in our lives. Also, virtually everyone has had the experience of looking through photographs in an album and bringing back memories of places, people and events which had been forgotten, but which come flooding back into conscious awareness when they look at those pictures. Here we are utilising these universal experiences to enable the client to recall memories of life as a non-smoker.

If the client has told you that they *did* successfully quit smoking for at least two weeks – say, for three weeks, or two months, or four years – then it is time to access that powerful resource. So you continue:

"So I'd like you to take down the photo album which shows those wonderful three weeks/two months/four years in which Jeff/Sue did live as a healthy, happy, non-smoker. And just glance through that album now, look at those pictures and notice how good it was to wake up in the morning feeling fresh, to feel high energy flowing through mind and body, to look in the mirror and see his/her face fresh, young, healthy, energised, to be able to enjoy home life, working, socialising, solving problems."

Here you can add any specific memories the client has mentioned from their recollections of the non-smoking life. Then continue:

"And notice how good it was to enjoy that happy, healthy, non-smoking life for day after day, week after week, month after month, year after year."

Of course, this depends on the actual length of time that the person was living as an ex-smoker. If it was, for example, three weeks, then of course you just say "day after day, week after week".

Now if the client has not stopped smoking previously for at least two weeks, and has continued in the habit ever since becoming a regular smoker, then your goal is to use this same photo album metaphor to take the client back to a time before the habit began. Let us assume that the client started smoking at the age of fifteen. In that case, you go back to the passage above which finishes "… your unconscious mind has full access to all those images," and continue:

"So I'd like you now to take down that photo album which shows the early years of Jeff's/Sue's life, those wonderful fifteen years in which he/she lived as a healthy, happy non-smoker. Just glance through those photos and see him/her growing, learning, socialising, playing, enjoying family life, travelling, throughout childhood and the early teenage years, enjoying that life for day after day, week after week, month after month, year after year, never once even thinking about that habit because it meant nothing to him/her."

Then, whether the client is looking at a memory of a time after they had quit smoking or before they had started the habit, continue:

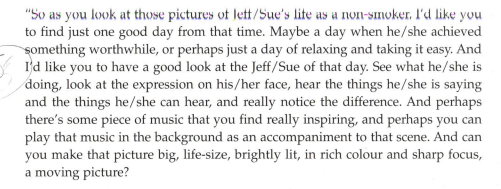

"So as you look at those pictures of Jeff/Sue's life as a non-smoker, I'd like you to find just one good day from that time. Maybe a day when he/she achieved something worthwhile, or perhaps just a day of relaxing and taking it easy. And I'd like you to have a good look at the Jeff/Sue of that day. See what he/she is doing, look at the expression on his/her face, hear the things he/she is saying and the things he/she can hear, and really notice the difference. And perhaps there's some piece of music that you find really inspiring, and perhaps you can play that music in the background as an accompaniment to that scene. And can you make that picture big, life-size, brightly lit, in rich colour and sharp focus, a moving picture?

"And if you like what you can see and hear, then I'd like you to step inside Jeff's/ Sue's body, so that you can feel the way your body feels, see what you can see with your own eyes, hear what you can hear with your own ears, perhaps continuing to hear that inspiring music. Actually live this life you're leading on this very good day, and really notice the difference. And say this affirmation to yourself: 'It's great to be a healthy, happy non-smoker. It's great to be a healthy, happy non-smoker." Say that in your own voice, in a confident, reassuring tone. Hear it on both sides of your head, as if it's in stereo, again and again and again."

As an alternative to the general affirmation contained in the above passage, you could substitute one based on the client's own words. For instance, if the client recalled that "I felt really proud of myself after I quit smoking," you could turn that into the following affirmation: "It's great to feel really proud of myself as a non-smoker." If a client remembers that "What was really good about being a non-smoker was the high energy I felt," then this could become: "It's good to feel such high energy as a non-smoker." The greater the utilisation of the client's own words, ideas and experiences, the more effective the entire process of hypnotherapy becomes.

What you have just asked the client to do is to look at the memory (the photograph in the album) from a *dissociated* standpoint. With dissociation, the client is standing *outside* of the picture looking at it. You also said that *perhaps* the client could hear a piece of music that they find inspiring to accompany that experience. If the client does indeed know of a particular piece of music that they already find inspiring, and may already associate with experiences of empowerment and achievement, then that piece of music is a powerful resource which you want to mobilise now in order to help the client become a non-smoker. On the other hand, if no such piece of music comes to mind, then you have retained rapport by using the word "perhaps". Whether the client experiences some inspiring music or not, they remain engaged with the process as what you have said is consistent with their experience.

Then you asked the client to step into that photograph and experience that same moment from an *associated* standpoint. With association, the client is experiencing, or remembering, that moment from *inside* their own body. An associated experience is more vivid and powerful than a dissociated one. At this point the client is maximally engaged with the experience. Now you are going to anchor this experience so that the client can retrieve it any time they feel the need for it. Continue:

"And if there's any word or phrase that comes into your mind that can describe this experience, then you can say that word or phrase out loud now if you like."

Listen carefully for the client's word or phrase. It could be "free", "happy", "alive with energy", or any number of others. If the client does say a word or phrase, then you repeat it out loud followed by the word "excellent". So if the client says, "Alive with energy", you reply:

"Alive with energy. Excellent. And in a moment, as you continue to see and hear and feel that experience, I'm going to touch your left wrist."

At this point, you establish an anchor for the positive memory which the client is experiencing in the moment. My preferred method is to firmly touch the client's left wrist while repeating a word which the client has provided. If you are going to touch the client, it is essential to let them know beforehand. However, if you have another method for establishing an anchor, then by all means use it.

While establishing the kinesthetic anchor, repeat the client's word or phrase again and again, with intensity in your voice. "Alive with energy, alive with energy, alive with energy." Then remove your hand from the client's wrist.

If the client simply remains silent in response to your request for a word or phrase, then that is fine. It could be that the client is already in a fairly deep trance and does not want to speak, or that they are simply remembering the sensory experience without any specific word or phrase coming to mind. From your point of view, it does not really matter. Remember that you said "… you can say that word or phrase out loud now if you like," thus validating the client's response, whether they say anything or not. Your task now is to validate the client and provide your own word as an anchor. If the client remains silent for three seconds, simply say:

> "Or you can simply enjoy that experience without putting a label on it at all. And in a moment, as you continue to see and hear and feel that experience, I'm going to touch your left wrist."

Then, as above, you touch the client's left wrist and provide a word or phrase as an anchor.

Some clients may ask for an explanation of the kinesthetic and auditory anchor you set up when you press their wrist and say a word or phrase while the client recalled the positive experience of living as a non-smoker. Explain:

> "What we did there was to set up what is called an anchor. Have you ever had the experience of hearing a piece of music that was in the charts ten years ago, but you haven't heard much since then, and as soon as you hear it, it brings back memories of people, places and situations from the time when that number was popular? Or maybe you can recall rummaging through an old trunk in an attic and coming across a forgotten object, and as soon as you pick it up, you see and hear and feel a flood of experiences associated with that object?

> "What we did with setting up that anchor is to get control over that process and make it available to you any time you want it. Your experience of life as a healthy, happy non-smoker already is there, stored inside, so any time you want to bring back that positive experience, all you need to do is to touch your wrist at that same point and say that word to yourself again and again."

If the client has already given you a word or phrase to describe their memory of the experience of being a non-smoker earlier in the session (for example, "cleaner", "more alert", or "a sense of achievement"), then use that word or phrase. If the client has not provided any such word or phrase, then the word "healthy" is likely to be accepted by all clients. So as you touch the client's wrist, you say the chosen word again and again: "Cleaner, cleaner, cleaner", or "Healthy, healthy, healthy".

Whether you have used your own or the client's word or phrase, you continue:

"And every time you want to re-experience this same very good day, all you have to do is touch your wrist at the same place and repeat that word/phrase to yourself again and again, and you'll experience it just as vividly as you are right now.

"And then I'd like you to step out of that experience, and this time take down that photo album which shows Jeff's/Sue's future life, one month in the future, Jeff's/Sue's life on 17th June 2010." (Use the date a month from today, or else some significant date coming up about a month in the future, such as New Year's Eve, or some holiday or family event that the client may have already mentioned. We will use 17th June 2010 as an example.)

"And I'd like you to have a good look at the Jeff/Sue of 17th June 2010. See what he/she is doing, look at the expression on his/her face, notice the position of his/her body, and hear the things he/she can hear. And really notice the difference. And perhaps you can hear that same inspiring music in the background as an accompaniment to that scene. And if you like what you can see and hear, then step inside Jeff's/Sue's body on 17th June 2010, so that you can feel the way your body feels on that date, see the things you can see with your own eyes, hear the things you can hear, perhaps including that same inspiring music, and really notice the difference." (Pause for a moment.)

"And then I'd like you to imagine that you're floating backwards through all the different photos which show everything that Jeff/Sue has done throughout the past month which has enabled him/her to achieve that future that you've just experienced. And at an unconscious level, I'd like you to make all the necessary insights and learnings and understandings that can make that future a reality in your life. And then I'd like you to float back, float back to the 17th May 2010 [today's date], step inside your own body sitting in that chair, and in your own time, become awake and alert and refreshed, and allow your eyes to open."

Allow the client all the time they want in order to return to waking awareness. Once the client's eyes are open, you ask the client, "Can you tell me what you

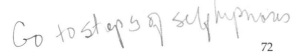

Go to steps 5 of self hypnosis

just experienced?" This is a general question which invites the client to describe what happened in their own words.

Remember that you've already said to the client at the beginning of the teaching of self-hypnosis that whatever they experience is authentic and that there is no right or wrong in any of this. So whatever the client says is consistent with this.

What you are particularly seeking from the client here is their description of memories of the past when they were a non-smoker, and representations of the future date that you have mentioned, both of which you have sought to elicit by use of the photo album metaphor. If the client does not give you these descriptions spontaneously in response to the general question, then ask more specifically: "Were you able to go back into your own past?"

Now some clients will not be able to directly access any memory of the non-smoking past at all. In that case, you say:

> "That's fine. Whatever you experience is correct and authentic for you. There's no right or wrong in any of this. That memory of your experience of living as a non-smoker is still in there, stored away at an unconscious level. In a few moments, we're going to ask the unconscious to draw on that memory and repeat that success."

With such clients, it is best not to ask about their experience of the future. Memories of the past are solidly grounded in real experience, while representations of the future – which has not happened yet – come from the imagination. If the client has not been able to access a memory of life as a non-smoker, then it is most unlikely that they will have been able to access a imaginary representation of the future. If you ask a client for a description of their internal experiences twice in a row, and get nothing to work with from the client's response both times, then it is likely that the client will start to lose confidence in the entire process. You can just about gloss over one blank response using the words above. However, with two such responses the whole session starts to fall apart.

Most clients, however, will remember at least something of the non-smoking experience via the photo album metaphor, whether distinctly or vaguely, and will give you a description of what they remembered. Listen to the client's answer and respond to it, and then continue:

> "Excellent. There are two purposes of that exercise. The first is to show how easy it is to create that state of relaxation any time you like. And if you can find those twenty minutes a day to practise doing this, then you'll find it a very useful way of cultivating the habit of relaxation. And the second purpose is to show that

the unconscious mind has representations of the future, just as it has memories of the past. You can bring back that sense of achievement/health [or whatever word or phrase was used in the anchor] any time you want it, just by touching your wrist in the same place and repeating that word/phrase. Were you able to go into your own future?"

Some clients will give you a description of a representation of the future. You then ask, "Were you aware of any cigarettes or smoking in that future?" If the client was able to access their representations of the future, then almost certainly they will answer "no".

You then respond,

"Excellent. Just as the unconscious mind has memories of the past, so too it has representations of the future. The great news is that as far as the unconscious mind is concerned, that *is* your future. In a moment, we're going to ask the unconscious mind to find the best, the most powerful way to make that future a reality in your life."

In a tiny number of cases, the client will experience a representation of the future in which they are still smoking. In order to deal with this very rare situation, once the client describes such an experience, you say:

"Yes. Right now your unconscious thinks of that future as a being a smoking one. But that representation of the future is an invention of the imagination – the future hasn't happened yet. What we're going to do in a few moments is to ask that creative part of your imagination, the unconscious mind, to find a way to change that future and make it a non-smoking one."

If the client was not able to access any representation of the future, then say,

"That's fine. The future hasn't actually happened yet, so it's not always easy to access it. But what we're going to do in a few moments is to ask your unconscious mind to create that future, drawing on the resources of your successful previous life as a non-smoker."

The five essentials of instant self-hypnosis

Some of your clients will take to self-hypnosis easily and effortlessly and be able to go along with everything you suggest. Others will have difficulty with some or all of the exercises. However, if they go along with the initial process of inducing instant self-hypnosis, you have achieved the minimum the exercise is for. The five essential steps to inducing instant self-hypnosis are:

(1) Close your eyes.
(2) Breathe slowly, deeply and evenly, from the diaphragm.
(3) Expel all the air from the lungs and breathe in new air.
(4) Say the word "calm" to yourself, silently and mentally.
(5) See the word "calm" written in front of you.

You can check by observation that the client is actually carrying out numbers 1, 2 and 3. Numbers 4 and 5 are so simple that anyone can do them. There are three main purposes of this section of the hypnotherapy session. Firstly (openly stated) is to show the client how they can create relaxation any time they want it. Secondly (not openly stated) is to induce a light trance state early in the session, so that later when you carry out the main induction, the client will go significantly deeper as a result of *fractionation*. With fractionation, the subject is repeatedly put into and awakened from trance. With each successive return to trance, the subject experiences a progressively deeper (more dissociated) state. Thirdly (not openly stated) is to remove any trepidation the client may have had about the prospect of experiencing hypnosis.

Self-hypnosis combined with stress management

The above is the way to teach self-hypnosis when the client does not mention stress as being an issue which leads them to smoke a cigarette. What follows is how to teach self-hypnosis when the client *does* mention the challenge of stress in their daily life. If the client is using cigarette-smoking as a form of stress management, then your task is to teach them a more useful way of managing that stress. I call this technique rapid variable stress management.

Validate the client by saying:

"A lot of people think that. They say, 'I feel stressed, I smoke a cigarette, it calms me down'. In fact, it's not the cigarette itself that calms a person down; indeed, the nicotine is actually a stimulant. But when a person experiences a situation, responds to it with stress and smokes a cigarette, three things happen.

"First of all, there's a shift of attention away from the situation which we've responded to with stress. Instead of being focused on that situation which we've responded to by creating stress, we're focused on fiddling about with the lighter, the cigarette, the ash, the ashtray, the whole business of lighting up and smoking. Because people often have to go outside to smoke these days, there can also be a physical move away from the situation where the experience of stress has taken place.

"Second, when the person inhales, it's that deep breathing that causes the mind and body to relax.

"Third, it can bring back memories of relaxed times with friends when cigarettes were being handed round.

"What we're going to do in a moment is a simple technique called instant self-hypnosis, which is a way of putting yourself into a peaceful, calm, relaxed, resourceful state any time you like, and it's much more useful than those cigarettes ever were in the past.

"What we're going to do is bring in what's called the relaxation response. Typically, when people undergo stress, they're experiencing what we call the 'flight or fight' syndrome. This is something we've inherited from prehistoric times. When a caveman/woman [if the client is male, use "man", if female, use "woman"] faced a hostile tribe or a sabre-toothed tiger or a woolly mammoth, he/she would experience the 'flight or fight' syndrome. What this meant is that the adrenalin would flow through the body, the muscles would be greatly strengthened, the heart would beat much more quickly, and the person could either fight with greater strength or else run away more quickly – the 'flight or fight' syndrome. Now the 'flight or fight' syndrome was very useful in prehistoric times, but because we've inherited it, every time we experience stress, the 'flight or fight' response kicks in as the best response we actually have available. Now, nature has also provided us with the opposite of the 'flight or fight' response, which is the relaxation response. This is where the muscles relax, the heartbeat and circulation slow, and the whole body and mind enter a peaceful, calm state. We can bring this about through instant self-hypnosis. It's very useful to do this for general health maintenance, quite apart from the specific issue we're here to deal with.

"Stress is neither good nor bad in itself. It's a bit like temperature. Sometimes it's desirable to be hot, sometimes we want to make ourselves cold, but we want to be in charge of that process and know how to make ourselves hot or cold.

"It's useful to think of stress as a numerical scale of alertness and relaxation between 100 and zero, in which 100 is the most severe stress it's possible to experience, and zero is absolute relaxation, like one of those holidays where we really don't need to do anything at all, in which all the muscles are completely loose, and there isn't even any thought, because we think with the muscles. A relaxed experience where we lose track of time and place.

"Now there is no absolute right or wrong on that numerical scale. Every number on that scale is useful and appropriate in some situation. Let's say someone's trapped under the wheels of a car. A bystander experiences exceptionally high stress; the adrenalin flows through the body. Their muscles become so strong that they can lift up the front of that car and release that person. At that point they're at 100 on that scale – but in that particular context, that's the most useful number on that scale to be at. But most of the time it's best to stay below 50 on that scale.

"Typically, people tend to push themselves higher up that scale than is really most appropriate for the situation they're in. What we need to do is have a way to always be able to find the most appropriate number on that scale for the par-ticular situation we're in. If it's a particularly busy day at work/dealing with the kids/etc" (obviously this depends on what the client's daily routine is), "you want an unusually high level of energy, stamina and adrenalin, so you might want to be at 40. If it's just an ordinary working day/day at home, then you would want to be at 30. If it's a pleasant relaxing evening with friends, one of those social occasions where the conversation flows freely, where you're interact-ing with those people, listening to them, talking to them, then you'd want to be at 20. If it's an experience of total relaxation, where all your muscles are relaxed, where you don't need to make conversation with anyone, or prove anything, where you can just lose track of time and place, then you might be at 5, or 3, or zero. But you want to be the one who decides where you go on that scale."

At this point, you train the client in instant self-hypnosis, just as in the simpler version described above. In the same way, you ask the client to adopt the cor-rect posture and breathing, and continue:

"Now with your *eyes closed*, I'd like you to focus on your breathing. Breathe slowly, deeply and evenly, building a nice, natural rhythm of deep, easy breathing."

In the above, verbally mark the words "eyes closed" by speaking them slowly and with greater emphasis. Verbal marking means saying certain words in a sentence in a particular way which distinguishes them from the others in the sentence. The goal is that the subject will respond to those marked words as a phrase in their own right. Continue:

"That's right. And the best place to breathe from is your diaphragm, which is just below your lungs, where your abdomen is, as you probably already know. And as you're breathing from the diaphragm, so your stomach is going up and down, and that's just fine, because it means that oxygen is flowing to every part of the body, which is exactly what the body needs. Good. And every time you breathe out, can you expel all the air from your lungs, breathing in completely new air, so that you're getting a really good air circulation. That's right. And every time you breathe out, in your own mind, say the word "calm" to yourself, silently and mentally. And every time you breathe out, see the word "calm", written right in front of you, written in your mind's eye. Good. And every time you do this, you'll be putting yourself into a peaceful, calm, comfortable state. And if you can find twenty minutes a day to practise doing this, maybe first thing in the morning, during some break in the day, perhaps when you come home in the evening, or maybe last thing at night" (depending on the client's routine), "then you'll be training your body in the habit of relaxation, which will have excellent long-term health benefits for you.

"And as you continue to enjoy this experience of instant self-hypnosis, you can be aware that everything you experience is authentic, there's no right or wrong in any of this.

"And be aware now that in this very relaxed state, your unconscious mind has access to all of your memories, stored away in the back of your mind. Something like photographs in a pile of albums, stretching way back over the course of your life. Big blow-ups and small prints, colour pictures and black-and-white, digital prints and Polaroids, thousands of photos showing every moment throughout the course of your life. And your unconscious mind has full access to all those pictures, all those memories.

"And the great thing is that you have already successfully found the most appropriate level of alertness and relaxation for each of the situations that you face in daily life. I'd like you to take down now that photo album which shows all of the photos of Jeff/Sue in the course of his/her working life. The great news is that there have already been many days throughout your career when you have successfully found just the right level of alertness and relaxation that is most useful for that particular situation.

"So I'd like you to glance through that album now and find just one unusually busy working day. A day where there was great deal of work to get through, to a tight deadline. A particularly demanding day when Jeff/Sue successfully found just the right level of alertness and relaxation to provide that energy, that stamina, that adrenalin, that he/she needed to get through that day. And when you've found that picture of Jeff/Sue successfully coping with that unusually busy day, have a good look at the Jeff/Sue of that day. Look at the expression on his/her face, notice how he/she holds his/her body, hear the tone of his/her voice and the things he/she is saying. Really examine that photo of Jeff/Sue successfully dealing with that very demanding day. And notice the number 40 in the top left hand corner of that picture, indicating 40 on that numerical scale. And if you like what you can see and hear, then I'd like you to step inside Jeff's/Sue's body in that picture, so that you can feel the way your body feels, see the things you can see with your own eyes and hear what you can hear with your own ears. And as you experience that, say that number 40 to yourself again and again and again. And see that number 40 written right in front of you. Forty, forty, forty, forty. And any time you want to re-experience just this level of alertness for any future busy day, all you have to do is say that number over and over again and you'll experience it just as vividly as you're aware of it right now.

"And now I'd like you to step out of that photo, and now flick through that album again, and I'd like you to find a picture of Jeff/Sue on an ordinary working day. A day which is neither particularly busy nor particularly slack. A day when Jeff/Sue found just the right level of energy and alertness and relaxation to get through that day. So when you've found that photo, have a good look at the Jeff/Sue of that day. Look at the expression on his/her face and the way he/she holds his/her body. Hear the things he/she is saying and the sound of his/her voice. Really notice the difference. And notice the number 30 in the top left hand corner of that photograph, indicating 30 on that numerical scale. So step inside Jeff's/Sue's body in that picture and feel the way your body feels on that ordinary working day, see what you can see with your own eyes and hear what you can hear, and really aware of the difference. And now say that number 30 to yourself again and again. And at the same time, see that number written right in front of you in huge numerals. Thirty, thirty, thirty, thirty. And every time you want to re-experience this same level of alertness and relaxation for an ordinary working day, just say that number to yourself and see that number, and you will experience it just the way you're feeling it right now.

"All right. So now I'd like you to step out of that photo and put that album of Jeff's/Sue's working life back on the shelf. And take down now that photo album which shows all of Jeff's/Sue's experiences of leisure time, down time, all those relaxing moments when Jeff/Sue has moved way down that numerical scale. So flick through that album now and have a good look through those relaxed experiences. And I'd like you to find a picture of an enjoyable social occasion, maybe one of those pleasant evenings with friends where the conversation just flows freely, and you even lose track of the passage of time. A fun time when you're actively engaged with those people, talking to them and listening to what they're saying. Have a good look at the Jeff/Sue in that picture now. Notice the expression on his/her face, the position of his/her body, listen to the tone of his/her voice and the things he/she is saying. And notice that number 20 in the top left hand corner of that photo. And if you like what you can see and hear, then step inside Jeff's/Sue's body in that picture, so that you can feel the way your body feels in that relaxed social occasion, see those people talking and joking, hear them speaking and laughing. And really notice the difference. And now say that number 20 to yourself again and again and again. Twenty, twenty, twenty. And at the same time see that number displayed right before your eyes. Twenty, twenty, twenty. And whenever you want to wind down and bring back this very same experience, all you need to do is see that number and say it to yourself just the way you're doing right now, and you'll experience it just as vividly as you're aware of it right now.

"So now step outside of that picture again, and this time, flick through that photo album and find the most relaxed experience of them all. A day of complete winding down, calmness, tranquillity. Maybe one of those holidays where you don't need to prove anything or even make conversation with anyone, where you can just enjoy the moment in the moment, or perhaps just a day of taking it easy at home, or maybe you'll find some other experience just like that. And when you've found that picture, take a good look at Jeff/Sue in that moment. See the expression on Jeff's/Sue's face, the position of his/her body. Notice the breathing. Hear the sounds in that environment. And notice that very low number in the top left hand corner of that photo. What number do you see?"

The client might reply, for example, "ten", "three" or "zero," or make no reply at all. If the client says a number, then use that number instead of the words "that very low number" in the passages below. If the client says nothing, then after three seconds say, "You can just look at that number without needing to say it out loud at all." Then you continue:

"So now, if you like what you can see and hear, then step inside Jeff's/Sue's body in that picture so that you can feel the way your body feels on that most pleasant and relaxed day. See what you can see and hear what you can hear. Just let yourself experience how good it is when you lose track of time, and your mind wanders freely. And say that very low number to yourself again and again, see that very low number right in front of you, and you know that every time you want to bring back this same experience, all you need to do is say that number and see that number and you'll bring back just what you're aware of right now." (Pause.)

"And now we'll do a simple exercise, just to ensure that you can always shift gear to bring back just the appropriate level of alertness and relaxation for every situation you will be facing in daily life. I'd just like you to imagine that you're driving along a beautiful, deserted country lane on a warm day in springtime, surrounded by the green of hedgerows and grass and leaves, and the blossom on the trees, with the sounds of birds singing. You already know about driving. About how you need to shift gear to adjust to different driving situations. So that when you're at top speed on the motorway, you're in fourth or fifth gear, and when you're driving through a town, you go into third, and when you turn a corner you go down to second, and when you're crawling along in heavy traffic or completely stationary, you go down to first. Well, as you drive along that country lane, I'd just like you to imagine that underneath your hand is a gear stick. But instead of the usual gears, there are the numbers 40, 30, 20 and that very low number – corresponding to those different numbers on that numerical scale. And when you shift to any of those numbers, so you can bring back that experience which corresponds to that same number.

"So now shift that gear stick right up to 40, and really notice how you can bring back that stamina and energy you need for that unusually busy day." (Short pause.) "Then move that stick down to 30, and be aware of that level of alertness and relaxation you need for an ordinary working day." (Short pause.) "And pull that stick down now to 20, so that you can just experience that pleasant social occasion, relaxed and enjoying that event. See that number 20, hear that number 20 again and again." (Pause.) "And now down to that very low number, and really let that very peaceful, tranquil moment flow through you. That's right." (Pause.)

"And now, just to make sure you've got the hang of it, move up to 20 again. Just experience that number. Feel it, see it, and hear it. That's right." (Pause.) "So now shift up to 30 – that ordinary working day – that's it, just to be aware of the difference." (Short pause.) "And now move up to 40 – just for a brief moment – just to know that, when you really need to, you can access that high level of stamina and adrenalin. And now down to 20 again. Seeing that number 20 and hearing it again and again. And then pull down once more to that very low number and really enjoy that experience for a few moments – until – in your own time – you can come back to the here and now, become awake and alert and refreshed and allow your eyes to open."

After the client has returned to full waking awareness, ask them, "So, how did you find that little exercise?" The client will then give you a description of their subjective experiences of self-hypnosis. If the client tells you that the exercise was easy to master as a means of accessing different stress levels for different situations, you know that it has been a success. If the client mentions any difficulty with it, or expresses doubt about their ability to repeat the process in everyday life, then work with the client until they have thoroughly mastered the technique and know that they can repeat it in future situations.

Preparing the client to stay a non-smoker in all situations

Every client is a unique individual. Different clients need help with specific issues, depending on their particular requirements. The hypnotherapist's task is to ensure that the client knows exactly how to stay a non-smoker in all situations after the session. Also, the hypnotherapist has to educate the client in techniques to ensure that they have control over any issue which is of particular concern to the individual, such as avoiding putting on weight or having a more useful way of focusing attention. You continue:

"We want to make sure that you stay a non-smoker in all situations, and self-hypnosis can be very useful in doing this. There are three main situations that you have to be prepared for in order to remain a non-smoker. The first is meeting an old friend. In that situation, the person who's a non-smoker maybe hasn't seen that friend for five years. They were always smoking together, and smoking was part of their friendship. The temptation might be there to have 'just the one' cigarette 'for old time's sake'. The problem is that the body doesn't understand the concept of 'just the one' cigarette. It understands two things: smoking and non-smoking. There's no 'middle way' or 'part-time smoking' or 'being a social smoker'. When the body experiences that nicotine coming in, it takes that as a signal: 'Oh, right, we must be going back to smoking mode again.' It's just like flipping a switch. Immediately the body reverts to its memory of those years of life as a smoker: pretty soon it's demanding five/ten/twenty cigarettes a day" (whatever number the client has been smoking recently). "So it's essential to avoid 'just the one' cigarette.

"The second situation is a difficult time in life, when the person might say, 'I'm just going to have one cigarette to get through this.' Then they're giving themselves the worst of both worlds. Smoking that cigarette puts them back on regular smoking again, and of course it's made no difference to the actual situation.

"The third situation is some social event, maybe someone's wedding or birthday, some celebratory dinner or function, or even just drinking with friends. The person's enjoying that occasion, they see others lighting cigarettes and offering them around, and they can think, 'Well, I'll just have one cigarette to enjoy this.' Of course, if they do that, then the habit continues long after the event has finished.

"So the thing to do – if you know that an event like that is coming up – is to prepare yourself for it through self-hypnosis. If you know you're going to be meeting an old friend who's still stuck with that habit, then put yourself in that relaxed state and just imagine meeting the old friend, enjoying the old friend's company, having a great time, but you remaining a non-smoker all the way through. See it, hear it and feel it in your imagination, as if you are an actor preparing for a part. So that when you actually meet the old friend, you can enjoy that experience and stay a non-smoker, even if the friend is chain-smoking all the way through.

"And if it's a difficult time in life, then put yourself in that same relaxed state and ask yourself these questions: 'How can I solve this?' 'How am I successfully dealing with this?' 'What's the answer to this?' As you ask yourself those questions, your unconscious mind will come up with answers, ideas, solutions that you can put into practice. A lot of people, when they face an unexpected difficulty, ask themselves, 'Why can't I solve this?' 'Why am I no good at dealing with this kind of situation?' The problem with saying that is that it tends to cut off the possibility of a solution because it presupposes that 'I can't solve this' and that 'I'm no good at dealing with this.' Unless we live in a cave in Nepal, we all face unexpected situations, often as a result of things which are not under our direct control, such as the actions of other people, or economic downturns and upturns. But we can control our *response* to those situations. And using self-hypnosis, we can tap into our inner resourcefulness and create the most useful response for every situation. And it's a lot better than simply reaching for a cigarette.

"When it's a social event coming up, the thing to do is to psychologically prepare yourself for it as a part of the whole routine of getting ready to go out. Just put yourself into that relaxed state and let yourself imagine what it would be like – going to the big party, having a great time, joking and laughing with those people, but you staying a non-smoker even if others are lighting up and offering cigarettes around. See it and hear it and feel it vividly in your imagination, and your unconscious mind will turn that into your reality. And this is the way to *stay a non-smoker* in all situations.

"One thing to be prepared for, now that you're becoming a non-smoker, is a situation in which one person among a group of friends has stopped smoking, but the others are still stuck in that habit. There can be a situation in which there's a kind of envy on the part of the others in the group. It's all done as a great big joke, but they can be offering cigarettes to the non-smoker, saying things like, 'Oh, go on, just have one, it won't kill you' or, 'We'll have you back on them by eleven o'clock tonight.' There's many a true word spoken in jest. Behind the big joke is the envy on the part of the smokers of the person who's become a non-smoker. 'Who does he/she think he/she is – does he/she think he/she's better than us or something?'" (Of course, use the client's own gender here.) "There's a desire to bring the non-smoker down to the level of the group. Or it could just be someone who thinks that they're being friendly or polite by offering a cigarette.

"Either way, there's a moment of temptation. And all you have to do is take a decision for that moment. You can add up all the incredible benefits you're enjoying now that you're a non-smoker – the much longer life, the better health, the greater energy, the easier breathing, the social advantages, the money you save, the sense of freedom" (at this point put one hand about two feet above the other, as if demonstrating a tall pile of benefits) "against maybe ten minutes of dubious pleasure by accepting that cigarette," (at this point hold up your finger and thumb with their tips very close to each other, as if demonstrating something very small) "and you'll make the correct choice" (putting one hand about two feet above the other, as before – non-verbal communication in action).

"Remember, you only have to take a decision for one moment. 'For this moment, I'm choosing to be a non-smoker.' It doesn't matter about next week, or tomorrow, or an hour from now, or even five minutes from now – for this moment I'm *choosing* to be a non-smoker.' So you just say, 'No thanks, I don't smoke' [with a gesture of rejection], the conversation moves on, and a few minutes later you'll have forgotten that moment. It takes twenty-one repetitions of an action to become a habit, and once you do that twenty-one times – 'No thanks, I don't smoke' [with the gesture] – it becomes a habit. You don't need to think about it. And this is the way to stay a non-smoker permanently."

The weight issue

A significant proportion of your clients – mostly, but not entirely, female clients – will express concerns about putting on weight when they stop smoking. Your task is to reassure them that they can become or remain just as slim as they want to be once they stop smoking, with factual information and a simple but effective action plan for getting control over their weight and eating habits.

If your client mentions concerns over their weight, you say:

"Sure. There are several reasons why people in some cases put on weight when they stop smoking. First of all, every cigarette contains sugar. This is partly a result of the production process, but sugar is also added. The reason why the manufacturers add sugar is to make cigarettes attractive to young smokers and because it builds up a sugar habit in the smoker, in addition to the nicotine habit. So when a person stops smoking, the body has got used to all that extra unnecessary sugar coming in many times a day, and suddenly it's not there any more, so the body expresses this incredible desire for sugary foods. Therefore when the ex-smoker eats the sweets, ice-cream, cakes, chocolate and other sugar-rich foods, the person is likely to put on weight. Also, there's a film of tar on the top of every smoker's tongue that dulls the taste buds. As the body clears itself of poison, that film of tar disappears, and we taste the food much more directly, so it tastes much better. In fact, as the body clears itself out, we get much more in touch with all the body's feelings, including the sensation of hunger. Even though the sensation of hunger is the same, we feel it more vividly, so we assume we must be more hungry than we really are, so we tend to eat more. Also, it can be a question of energy. That smoking habit has consumed a lot of energy, and when a person stops smoking, there can be the temptation to pick at a nice piece of cheese here, a nice bit of cake there [miming the actions of picking at food]. What we want to do is to find a more useful outlet for that energy.

"In order to become or remain slim, we have to give the body what it really needs. The human body is 70 percent water, so the body needs primarily water-rich foods to sustain itself. This includes fresh fruit, fresh vegetables, salads, fruit juice, water itself. There's a Chinese saying: 'Eat food which perishes quickly – but eat it before it perishes.' That's very useful advice to follow. If food perishes quickly, that means that it's close to nature, and the bacteria love it. But the more food is processed, the less nutritional value it has. Sure, it lasts longer, but that's because the bacteria won't touch it. So in order to remain slim, water-rich foods should be the main part of what you eat."

Many clients will have a particular food that they enjoy which is not exactly consistent with slimness when eaten to excess. Examples include cheese, chocolate, bread, cakes, ice cream and salami. In such cases, your goal is to show the client that they do not need to completely give up that food. Rather, they can learn to look on it as a special treat to be enjoyed, say, once a week. You advise the client to go to a small high-priced shop in their locality which specialises in selling the desired food, and to buy a small quantity of a luxurious, expensive, high-quality example of the food concerned. Then, having paid an exorbitant price, the client is to really focus their attention on enjoying every bite of the food, relishing every nuance of flavour, and making the most of it as the big treat of the week. The visit to the expensive shop can become something the client looks forward to every week. Thus the client will still be able to enjoy the particular food concerned, and will be able to avoid putting on weight without any sense of deprivation.

So if the client has a liking for cheese, for instance, you would say:

> "But no food is off limits. If you really enjoy eating cheese, then look on that as a treat. Maybe go to a very expensive deli or cheesemonger at the end of the week and buy a small piece of fine French or Italian cheese at an outrageously high price, and really enjoy every morsel of it. So that you're not depriving yourself of anything, but instead getting more pleasure out of less of that favourite food."

You continue by providing tips which enable the client to enjoy healthy food while remaining in control of their eating and thus avoiding weight gain. You say:

> "It's important to get in touch with your body's natural stomach hunger. Many people respond to mouth hunger. But your stomach will give you a signal that it's really hungry, and that's your cue to start eating. As far as possible, eat only at mealtimes. If you do want to snack, make sure that you have fruit available. You'll find that the sugar in the fruit will give you all the sugar you need. Fruit is nature's way of giving us a drink in a solid format – it's mainly liquid, but it can easily be carried around.

> "When you eat a meal, learn to eat like a gourmet. Eat only when you are really hungry – with that signal of stomach hunger. A gourmet looks at the food, enjoys the layout and presentation, smells the food and appreciates the aroma. A gourmet will tell you that 50 percent of the pleasure of the meal is enjoyment of the presentation. Then, in their own time, a gourmet will cut off a tiny mor-sel of food, look at it, smell it, put it in their mouth, chew it thoroughly, rolling it around every part of the tongue to get the full flavour, really noticing every nuance of flavour, then swallow it. Then they unhurriedly cut off another piece and do the same with that. And then when they get the signal from the stomach that it's full up, that's the signal to stop eating. Even if there's food left on the plate, that food goes in the fridge or in the bin – there's plenty more where that came from.

"Another useful way of enjoying less food while staying slim is to put the food on a smaller plate. It makes it look as if there's more food than there really is. Experiments have shown that people feel more full up after they've eaten the same amount of food from a smaller plate than a bigger one. This is true even when they themselves have measured the same amount of food onto a big and a small plate. Sure, it's only an optical illusion, but if it keeps you both slim and happy with the amount you've eaten, why not use it?

"And that's the way to stay as slim as a non-smoker."

The drinking issue

A significant proportion of clients mention drinking alcohol because they are concerned about "losing control" when they go out drinking with friends. Others will say that they are concerned about putting on weight as a result of their drinking, or substituting alcohol for the cigarettes they have given up. It could be a combination of these concerns. Either way, you give the client the information they need to know, together with comprehensible advice as to how to deal effectively with the drinking issue.

You say:

"A lot of people think that when they drink alcohol they somehow lose control and become a completely different person who is no longer in charge of their actions. Actually, this is more to do with our cultural expectations than with reality. There's an experiment in psychology where the experimenters gave one group of people a drink which they were told was an alcoholic cocktail but in fact contained no alcohol – it was just a mixture of fruit juices and syrup. The experimenters gave a second group of people a drink which *did* contain alcohol, but they told them, 'Oh, this is a non-alcoholic cocktail.' What was remarkable was that an hour later the group which *thought* that they had drunk the alcohol, but in fact had drunk the non-alcoholic drink, were slurring their speech, fooling around and generally acting drunk, while the group which *had* drunk the alcohol, but thought it was alcohol-free, continued exactly as they had before with no noticeable difference in their behaviour. So it's really about our expectations rather than reality.

"A good way of dealing with the whole question of alcohol is to make drink your friend. Learn to become a connoisseur of wine [whisky, beer, depending on the client's preference]. Make wine [or whatever] your friend. Get to know the different grapes, the regions, the countries, the vintages. Look on wine as a delicacy and a treat. Maybe go to an up-market wine merchant and buy some really expensive wine. Then when you drink the wine, drink like a connoisseur. A connoisseur looks at the colour of the wine in the light, smells it to get the aroma, sips it and rolls that sip all the way around the mouth, noticing every nuance of flavour. The true connoisseur doesn't even drink it – they spit it out. You don't quite need to go that far, but the point is to get more pleasure out of less drink by really focusing on it, enjoying it and looking on it as a treat. So you're getting more pleasure out of less alcohol. So maybe instead of drinking six glasses in an evening, you can get more pleasure out of one or two glasses, by drinking as a connoisseur. And remember, you remain the same person even after you've had a few drinks, and you can stay a non-smoker in all situations."

This approach is similar to that above for the client with a liking for a particular food. Of course, drinking alcohol can also be a cause of excess weight, so here you are helping the client in both ways.

Marijuana

A significant minority of clients who want to quit the tobacco habit smoke marijuana (cannabis, "pot", "dope", "weed", "hash", "ganga", "smoke"). In Britain, marijuana usually comes as "skunk," in the form of a solid block of hash. This is then mixed with tobacco and rolled into a joint. This is because the hash is extremely pungent and strong to taste. Now, if a person wants to stop smoking and stay stopped, they must avoid any exposure to tobacco. There are many people who successfully stop smoking for months or years, but then smoke a joint (containing both marijuana and tobacco) and instantly the body reverts to its desire for cigarettes, putting the person back on, say, twenty tobacco cigarettes a day.

In some cases, the client wishes to give up both tobacco and marijuana at the same time. This is by far the easiest and best option for both the client and the therapist. The two issues can easily be dealt with at the same time. In fact, it is far easier to stop smoking marijuana than it is to quit tobacco. Marijuana is far less habit-forming from a physical point of view. If the client wishes to quit both marijuana and tobacco in the same session, then for the most part you need to add the word "marijuana" to the word "tobacco". If your client mentions marijuana, you reframe and pace it just as with cigarettes. You could say:

"When a person smokes marijuana" (or "weed", "dope" or whatever word the client uses), "they do so for a reason. People want to find a way to change their mood. They can do this by smoking marijuana or some other illegal drug, drinking a glass of whisky, drinking tea or coffee, or taking some tablet prescribed by the doctor. When people smoke marijuana, they generally do it because getting stoned enables them to feel relaxed, mellow, creative, sociable. These are all positive and desirable experiences to have. The great news is that any mood or emotion we've experienced in the past from any kind of drug, we can bring back through self-hypnosis.

"So there are two possible ways forward. I would say that the best and easiest is to simply stop smoking marijuana as well as tobacco, and cultivate instead the habit of self-hypnosis, so that you can create that mood at will. It's a lot cheaper and you can always be sure of scoring a good supply. We want to make sure that you never inhale any tobacco in the future, whether it be from a cigarette or from a joint. Now the way it's usually done in the UK is to mix the joint using both marijuana and tobacco. And if you smoke it that way, then the moment your body tastes that tobacco coming in, it's going to revert to its smoking mode and demand five/ten/twenty cigarettes a day. So if you really do want to continue smoking marijuana, the thing to do is to smoke it American style. In the States, it comes in grass format and is smoked neat, without adding anything to it. If you can always make sure it's in grass format, and you never add any tobacco to it, then that is a possible way forward. But you must make sure that you never take even a puff of someone else's mixed joint. That would be the route back to smoking tobacco. So if you're going to some social event where there's likely to be joints handed round, then the thing to do is bring your own stash of grass and smoke only that – never anyone else's. And that *is* a way of staying a non-smoker of tobacco while still consuming marijuana. Which would you prefer to do?"

The client can then decide between the two alternatives. If the client chooses to give up marijuana altogether, then include suggestions for the cessation of smoking marijuana along with suggestions for quitting tobacco.

The same principle is applied with certain other illegal drugs. People snort cocaine and its derivatives in order to give themselves energy and a buzz and become more bubbly and talkative. In the same way, you can pace that desire and lead it, giving the client a more useful way of creating energy. However, with the case of heroin consumption, it is best to regard that as a separate issue, not to be dealt with in the same session as tobacco smoking cessation. If a client is habituated to both heroin and tobacco, let the client know that they will be better off as a non-smoker, and can achieve freedom from heroin at a later date.

Focusing attention

Some clients will tell you that they use the smoking habit as a means of focusing their attention on some task that they have to do, such as making an important phone call. In this case, the smoking habit fulfils a valuable function, and your task is to show the client a more useful way of achieving that function than smoking a cigarette. So you can tell the client this:

"Here's an exercise to focus your attention on some task you want to carry out, such as making a telephone call. In the days of the old silent films, they would use a 'key' to focus the audience's attention on one particular part of the scene.

The key would typically be a circle in which a person's face, or an object on the table, or something else of significance, was brightly lit, while everything else around that circle was in complete darkness. In the same way, in live theatre, if they want to focus the audience's attention on one person or object, they change the lighting from diffused floodlight to a single spotlight. What we are going to do now is use the same principle in the same way, so that the whole of your attention becomes focused on the task at hand.

"Typically, as we go through daily life, our thoughts are diffused: we are thinking about several different things, and all sorts of sounds and visual cues are competing for our attention. We need a way of focusing attention that is consistent with our long-term good health.

"Let's say you need to focus your attention on making a phone call. Sit looking at the desk with the phone on it in the centre of your vision. Then just imagine that there is a spotlight attached to the centre of your forehead. Something like a miner's helmet with a torch [flashlight in the US] attached to it. You can move that spotlight so that it's pointing anywhere you like. Shine that spotlight on the area of the desk in which the phone is the centre. Imagine that the spotlight creates a circle of light so that that area with the phone in the centre is brightly lit. Meanwhile, in your imagination, fade down the light in the area outside the circle, so that it becomes dark, then darker, then completely black. Turn down the volume of the sounds outside that circle, as if you were turning down the volume control on an imaginary CD player. Now your entire attention is focused on that phone and the call you have to make. Of course, you can adapt this technique to any and every situation."

Cravings

It is an odd fact that after the hypnotherapy session some clients will experience no cravings at all, while others do experience cravings. In principle, the hypnotherapeutic communication with the unconscious mind is supposed to bring about a complete transformation in which the body's cravings simply disappear. In practice it is not always quite as simple as that.

Many people experience some form of physical craving even after the hypnotherapy session. It is essential to prepare the client for either of these two future possibilities. In the case of a smoker who did stop before for at least two weeks, you say: "When you stopped smoking for six weeks/four months/two years [or whatever] before, did you experience any kind of cravings or withdrawal symptoms at the beginning of that period?" The client might say something like, "Yes, I felt irritable." Or the client might say, "No, I felt just fine" – which indicates that they became a non-smoker at an unconscious as well as a conscious level. Many clients have not stopped smoking before. In any event, it is essential to prepare the client for dealing with physical cravings after stopping smoking – even though ideally no such cravings will be experienced. Say:

"Sure. When a person stops smoking at a conscious level but has not dealt with the unconscious aspect of the habit, the body gets confused. For all those years it's adjusted to having five/ten/twenty (or whatever) doses of nicotine coming in every day. All of a sudden, there's nothing coming in. So the body gets confused. 'Hey, it's five o'clock in the afternoon – I haven't had a cigarette all day – what's going on?' Those physical cravings are the body expressing that confusion. But what we're doing today is dealing with the *unconscious* part of the mind. Once the unconscious knows that you're a non-smoker, it communicates that fact to every part of you, so that your body, too, knows that you are a non-smoker.

"Your body welcomes this breathing space that you're giving it and there shouldn't be any cravings at all. It takes about two weeks for the body to clear itself out of all the tar, nicotine and carbon monoxide that's stuck inside. It's a very powerful, very rapid transformation. Within eight hours from now, the amount of nicotine inside you will go down by half, your pulse and heartbeat will return to their healthy level. Over the next two weeks, your senses of smell and taste will come back to their proper level. Two weeks from now, the process will be complete. You can walk into a crowded room or bar which is filled with smoke, and if a waft of smoke comes up to your face, it will smell horrible, your eyes will water, you might want to cough – that's because your body's natural defence mechanisms have come back. They're saying, 'Hey, this is a poison – be wary of it.' And you can trust your body's defence mechanisms to protect you physically. It's also essential to make sure that you are psychologically well defended, so that you are prepared for any and every situation.

"Now we're dealing with the unconscious part of the mind, so there shouldn't be any cravings during that two-week cleansing process. But do bear in mind it's a massive physical transformation, and that you did experience those cravings when you stopped before," (obviously, you only say these words if they correspond to the client's experience) "so there may be the odd tweak as your body goes through that cleansing process again. Just remember that if you do experience anything like that, then it only lasts for ten seconds. If you can distract your mind for ten seconds, maybe drink a glass of water, eat an apple, read the paper, listen to the radio, just for ten seconds, then it will disappear, and if you do experience anything like that, then they'll become fewer and weaker over the next two weeks until they disappear completely. And remember that, even in the event that, during that two-week process of cleansing, any such cravings feel quite strong, do remember that nobody has ever died from allowing their body that breathing space."

Left unspoken is the fact that reverting to smoking can indeed cause death. You do not need to spell out that fact.

Transfer of energy

It is important to deal with the question of energy with your client. If the client has previously stopped smoking for more than two weeks, you ask, "When you became a non-smoker for those three months/two years, etc, before, how was your energy level?" The client might say something like, "Much better. I found it was easy to run upstairs." If the client does recall such an increase in energy, then you say, "Excellent. Now that you're becoming a non-smoker again, you'll recover that same level of energy." Or it could be that they recall no noticeable difference in energy levels. Other clients, of course, have not stopped smoking before.

Whether the client has a recollection of increased energy as a non-smoker or not, you say:

> "When a person stops smoking, they generally experience a significant increase in energy. That smoking habit has consumed a great deal of energy. Physical energy, because those five/ten/twenty doses of nicotine coming in every day are a heavy burden on the body. There's also a lot of work with the fingers – all the fiddling about with the lighter, cigarette, ashtray and ash. Also, if a person's smoking ten cigarettes a day, it means that the hand is going up to the mouth and down again a hundred times a day. That's an awful lot of energy – you could probably power the lights in this room off that amount of energy."

From a strictly scientific point of view, this assertion is probably an exaggeration. It is intended as an illustrative story, to get the client to realise that a great deal of energy has been consumed by the smoking habit, and that they will have to find a more useful outlet for that energy now that they are stopping smoking. The colourful story is likely to bring to the client's conscious mind recollections of seeing or hearing about actual devices in which bicycle pedals can be worked by human feet in order to power a set of light bulbs. These devices demonstrate the amount of energy that bodily action can produce. Continue:

> "Now when a person stops smoking for the first time, they experience a huge increase in energy. It can seem like manic energy or restlessness, but that's simply what non-smokers experience anyway. It's important to have a positive outlet for all that extra energy. I don't know if you do any sports, or have any hobbies or interests, but you might like to devote more energy to them. A good way of channelling all that energy in a useful direction is to get into the habit of walking. Walking is an excellent exercise because it uses all the muscles of the body. So maybe if you want to go and visit someone, or buy something, you might think, 'Yes, I could walk there and back, rather than driving or going by public transport.' So you can integrate that habit into your daily routine without having to make a great effort to go the gym, or the tennis court, or the golf

91

course. It's definitely something worth thinking about, how you're going to manage that energy."

You have now prepared your client for every possible situation they are likely to face in real everyday life after finishing the session. It is important when dealing with the above to bear in mind two factors.

First, you must ensure that the client's specific requirements have been properly dealt with. The client must fully understand the techniques and how to apply them in the everyday world. If the client comes up with some unexpected concern which is not addressed here, then the hypnotherapist should deal with that concern from the repertoire of techniques with which every effective hypnotherapist should be familiar.

Second, it is not enough merely to demonstrate these techniques in the session. Many, if not most, clients, will have difficulty in remembering the precise details of the techniques, so it is essential to give a written handout, and possibly also a CD, in which they are described in detail.

Chapter 7

The trance induction and after

Main trance induction

Now is the time to induce trance. Remember that the self-hypnosis exercise you taught the client early in the session means that the client has already experienced a trance state, even if only a light one. The consequence of the main trance induction is that the client will re-enter trance. (Therefore the client will experience fractionation as they are repeatedly put into and awakened from trance.) This second trance that you are about to induce is therefore likely to be deeper than the first, and – connected with this fact – any trepidation that the client may have had early on about entering trance has already been cleared away by their pleasant experience with self-hypnosis.

Inducing a deep trance does not necessarily of itself mean that the client will become a non-smoker. Some clients enter a very deep trance and are difficult to awaken, but go back to smoking within twenty-four hours of the session. Other clients who successfully stop smoking and stay stopped report that they were conscious of everything that the hypnotherapist said during the main induction and "didn't think they were hypnotised". It is the totality of the hypnotherapy process, from the prelude in which positive expectations for success are built up, to the completion of the session itself, and in many cases what happens after the session, which turns a smoker into a non-smoker.

At some point there will be a moment of transformation in which the unconscious part of the client's mind experiences an epiphany or breakthrough. This epiphany could conceivably occur before the session has even begun. For instance, if the hypnotherapist has successfully helped a friend, relative or work colleague of the client to stop smoking, they have an especially powerful expectation of success even before the "official" therapy starts. It is as though the client has become a non-smoker even before meeting the therapist. In others, the epiphany comes during the early stages of the session, when the therapist is teaching the client to gain control over their internal subjective experiences. Or it could happen while the therapist teaches the client to practise self-hypnosis, during the main induction, at the very end of the session, after the session or during a subsequent session. Because there is no way of knowing beforehand when this moment of transformation will happen, we have to maximise the effectiveness of every single element of the hypnotherapy session – not just the main induction.

Why induce trance at all? There are three reasons for this. First, it fulfils the client's expectations. The client expects to be hypnotised, and that is what they get. Second, it enables "communication without noise" to use William Kroger's phrase. Trance enables the message to get across without the noise that comes from the client's critical inner voice and thoughts about other matters. Third, closely connected to the above, it enables a mobilisation of the client's creative imagination – a faculty which can best be accessed in the noise-free environment of trance.

So what exactly is trance and how do we induce it? As mentioned above, the conscious mind is aware of only a very limited amount of information at any given moment; everything else is unconscious. Our task is to communicate effectively with the unconscious part of the mind by overloading or distracting the conscious mind. We have to shift the whole of the client's conscious attention to something which completely absorbs it, and then we can communicate with the client's unconscious mind without interference by the conscious mind.

To most clients, dissociation is the characteristic of hypnotic trance that they expect to experience in their session with you. Most clients assume that dissociation means that the hypnotic subject does not consciously hear what the hypnotist says. When hypnotherapists themselves talk about "deep trance", they generally mean that the client experiences dissociation. In other words, if during trance the client loses conscious awareness of what you are saying, then they will generally assume that they have been hypnotised, and therefore that the session is more likely to be successful than it would have been in the absence of dissociation. We know that if a client says, "But I heard everything you said," then that generally suggests a scepticism about whether they were in fact hypnotised and therefore uncertainty about whether the session was successful. The truth is that dissociation is neither essential to achieve success nor does it necessarily create success.

More important than achieving dissociation is getting the client fascinated and absorbed by the experience of hypnotic trance and in mobilising their creative imagination in order to find the solution to the smoking problem. The client is usually not interested in hypnosis as such. They are interested in becoming a non-smoker, and regard hypnosis as a means to an end. Therefore, do not talk much about hypnosis or hypnotic phenomena. Talk about the one subject that you can be certain every client is fascinated and absorbed by: himself or herself. The most reliable way to absorb your client's conscious awareness and induce an hypnotic trance is to talk about this perennially-fascinating subject.

In the early stages of the session, listen constantly for both information about the client that they voluntarily give, and for figures of speech, metaphors, catch-phrases and references which indicate something about how the client forms their model of the world. Also, be alert for descriptions of strategies by which they have achieved successful transformations in other areas, and if necessary ask for more details. For instance, if the client successfully trained for and completed a marathon, or if the client was an alcoholic and successfully gave up drinking, then the strategy they used to achieve that result could be utilised in trance. Ask, "How did you do that?" or, "What can you remember about that?" The information they give you can be fed back in trance by asking the unconscious to follow a proven strategy to achieve an similar success in becoming a non-smoker.

All the trance inductions that are taught at hypnotherapy schools will get some clients into trance at least some of the time. But the drawback of many of them is that they require the client to do a lot of work. Many induction techniques require the client to focus on two or more actions or thoughts at the same time, or they command the client to accept orders from the therapist, implying an authoritarian relationship. In most cases induction techniques get the client to do things the therapist's way, which means the client has to leave their comfort zone and do awkward and unfamiliar things. All too often one hears accounts from people who have been hypnotherapy clients of how "I didn't feel any different" and "I just sat there with my eyes closed while the hypnotist talked on and on."

To be certain that the client experiences a satisfactory trance state, it is best to use inductions which ensure that, as far as possible, the client remains in their comfort zone at all times and experiences thoughts, feelings and processes which are both familiar and pleasant. This maximises both the effectiveness of trance induction, and the client's own enjoyment of the experience.

The essence of effective hypnotic communication is to create a context in which the result you are seeking happens without you having to specify it. By way of example, consider this question: have you heard about Pavlov's experiments with dogs, in which he would ring a bell every time the dogs were served food, and then would ring the bell all by itself, without the food being served? And are you now salivating? If you are, that is because these words just created a context in which you salivated without even seeing a mention of the word. You already know about Pavlov's experiments with the dogs, the bell and the food, so that as you read these lines, your unconscious mind brings in the idea of salivating which is associated with them. Because we always relate what we hear to ourselves, your body responds by secreting saliva into the mouth. Yet the words "saliva" or "salivate" are not mentioned. Now read the words: "Salivate – I order you to salivate – you must salivate now." Are you now salivating? It's most doubtful. The drawback of making direct commands in this way is that the critical aspect of the conscious mind is aware of them and in fact it is quite difficult to make yourself salivate on command – certainly harder than creating a context in which it happens unconsciously.

This is the essence of what is often called "Ericksonian hypnotherapy". Milton Erickson was a psychiatrist who is best known for his remarkable innovations in the use of hypnosis in medical practice. After Erickson's death in 1980, the concept of Ericksonian hypnotherapy came into vogue as a result of the teaching of certain selected techniques from the later years of Erickson's life. A cottage industry emerged based on a selected part of Erickson's work, constructing something called Ericksonian hypnotherapy – which has subsequently taken on a life of its own.

Yet Erickson himself never used the term "Ericksonian hypnotherapy" in any of his published writings or seminars. As far as he was concerned, he was discussing hypnosis and how to use it most effectively. Perhaps the two key concepts which he emphasised as being most important to effective hypnosis were utilisation and tailoring – utilising what the client actually does and the resources they possess, and tailoring the entire therapeutic process to the specific individual. The term "Ericksonian hypnosis" has come to mean hypnotherapy that emphasises these two concepts.

Having said that, some of the fundamental concepts underpinning Ericksonian hypnotherapy are essential for the working hypnotherapist to understand, if they wish to ensure maximum success:

(1) the client already has the all the resources within them that are needed to achieve their goals;
(2) the therapist's task is to mobilise those resources in order to bring about an internal learning or reorganisation which results in the transformation the client seeks;
(3) the therapist does not know – nor does the client, at least at a conscious level – how precisely this internal learning or reorganisation will take place. Nor do they know which of a number of possible positive outcomes the unconscious mind might achieve;
(4) the therapist communicates with the client effectively by specifically tailoring the entire session to them, and by utilising the client's actions, words and experiences as tools to construct the therapy and to move the client forward in the desired direction. *Tailoring* and *utilisation* are effective forms of communication which achieve rapport and unconscious transformation.

These principles have been derived or modelled from a *part* of Erickson's vast body of work by other people, and are not necessarily the way Erickson would have expressed it. The therapist needs to know about them. However, relying solely on Ericksonian indirect, permissive and maternalistic hypnotic communications with smoking cessation can bring a result different from the desired one because of a phenomenon known as "smoker's logic". When a person is a smoker, even if they know the risks of smoking and express a desire to stop smoking at a conscious and intellectual level, nevertheless the unconscious mind, which has been keeping the smoking habit going all these years, will use any and every rationalisation – however ludicrous and absurd – to either stay smoking or to go back to that habit once the person has quit smoking for a short period of time.

It may be asked why, if the unconscious mind always does what it believes is in the person's best interest, so many people engage in what looks like self-damaging behaviour. The biologist Paul Martin provides part of the answer:

> "Smokers now acknowledge the unappetizing fact that their behaviour significantly increases their risk of dying prematurely from heart disease or cancer. Nevertheless, psychological research has established that they seriously underestimate the magnitude of that risk. There is a consistent 'optimistic distortion' of perceived health risks among smokers; they know smoking is bad for them but they do not recognize just *how* bad. No matter how often the statistics are quoted they do not seem to sink in. One reason why the health consequences of smoking have such a muted impact on people's perceptions is the large delay, often measured in decades, between starting to smoke and falling ill."[1]

Also, when people who have previously quit smoking revert to the habit, they usually do so while in a momentary state of heightened emotional arousal, whether positive or negative.

One young female client of mine stopped smoking after our session for several months. However, she then went on a very enjoyable holiday with a group of friends, most of whom were smokers. She recalled that during one particularly absorbing late-night after-dinner conversation, it struck her that all the interesting, trendy and clever people in the group were smoking. She accepted an offered cigarette, and immediately reverted to smoking.

Conversely, a businessman who came to see me stopped smoking for over a year after the session. Unfortunately, his company then went bankrupt, causing him substantial financial losses. Within minutes of receiving official notification of that fact, he lit a cigarette and returned to the smoking habit.

The "left-brain" mental world of Aristotelian logic, of causality, of mathematical calculations, governs science and technology. The "right-brain" world, by contrast, makes sense of reality through "irrational" metaphorical associations. My view is that in such a moment of heightened emotional arousal, the person enters a form of trance in which thought, feeling and action respond to "right-brain" processes and bypass the critical faculty in the immediate situation.

The female client referred to above formed a momentary association between "interesting, trendy and clever people", and smoking. In that moment of positive emotional arousal, the unconscious mind uncritically accepted the idea that smokers are "interesting, trendy and clever" people, and therefore she smoked a cigarette.

With the client who returned to smoking when his business collapsed, in the emotionally aroused (negative) state he was in when he heard that news, it is likely that he sought immediate comfort. For many years before he had quit the habit, a cigarette had been a way of attaining comfort in unpleasant and difficult situations. He had undoubtedly established many pleasant anchors connected with smoking during those years: memories of experiences such as relaxed social occasions with friends, celebrating successes and enjoying a reflective moment to himself. In that momentary state, he smoked a cigarette as an immediately-available means of achieving those desirable associations, without challenge by the critical faculty.

The rationalisations which smokers provide in explaining why they reverted to the habit is often worthy of the delightful pseudo-logic of the Cheshire Cat, Humpty Dumpty and the Red Queen in Lewis Carroll's stories. One young lady client of mine said that she *had* stopped smoking. However, after a non-smoking friend of hers died of a brain haemorrhage at the age of 33, she decided to go back to smoking. She took the view that if her friend had died young despite being a non-smoker, she (the client) may as well go back to smoking, as her prospects could hardly be any worse as a smoker!

So the problem with using exclusively Ericksonian communications, in which the client's unconscious is encouraged to come up with any number of possible future outcomes, is that the unconscious is likely to come up with an absolutely wonderful creative process of inner transformation … in which the client remains a smoker.

Therefore to bring about successful smoking cessation, we need to supplement the Ericksonian style of communication with direct, authoritarian and paternalistic commands in which the therapist tells the client that they are to stop smoking and stay stopped, with no possibility of misinterpretation or of multiple possible outcomes from that point of view.

The therapist is using a technique which is reminiscent of the "good cop, bad cop" approach used by the police when they want to get information or a confession out of a suspect held in custody. One officer (the "good cop") communicates to the suspect in a friendly and sympathetic manner, talking about the possible benefits of cooperating with the police, and even coming across as seeming to be on the side of the suspect. Then the other ("the bad cop") enters and interrogates the prisoner in a hostile, aggressive and humiliating manner, threatening to prosecute him for numerous offences and impose exceptionally severe penalties. The bad cop walks out and the good cop takes over again, encouraging the suspect to vent his anger about the bad cop's approach and encouraging the suspect to be reasonable, holding out the hope of a compromise on charges if the suspect will give the police what they want. The technique is probably as old as policing itself, and it works remarkably well.

By analogy, the therapist using hypnosis for smoking cessation needs to switch from an Ericksonian permissive, indirect and maternalistic approach to a more directive, authoritarian approach – telling the client unambiguously to become a non-smoker. Both approaches draw on the client's internal resources. With the "permissive" side, you are invoking their creative imagination, ability to learn and previous experience of living as a non-smoker, and with the "authoritarian" side, you are drawing on the many years of propaganda and nagging against smoking that the client has been subjected to, and also their conscious decision to become a non-smoker. With smoking cessation, hypnotic communication is most effective when it combines both direct and indirect approaches. Direct, so that there is a clear and unambiguous goal as to the positive outcome to which the client is supposed to be headed. Indirect, so as to enable the client's creative imagination to find their own unique route to that positive outcome.

Relationships of power and status

All communication takes place in a context. If a doctor of medicine tells a patient to do something, the patient does it without engaging in a debate, without asking critical questions or answering back. It is an unequal relationship in which the power, prestige and knowledge rests mostly with the doctor. The patient accepts the nature of this relationship, and any communications made within this context is likely to reflect that. For example, when a doctor tells a patient under their care, "You've got to stop smoking", four percent of patients stop smoking the instant the doctor says those words. By contrast, if a lay hypnotherapist, who has never seen the inside of a medical school, were to say, "You've got to stop smoking. That's £200, please," then one suspects that the client might consider that they were being overcharged – and quite rightly so.

The key question to ask yourself is this: what is the most useful communication I can possibly convey to this particular client in this particular moment for this particular purpose we are both aiming to achieve?

The most effective trance inductions

We will now examine how to induce trance reliably, followed by an exploration of what to actually say to the client once a satisfactory trance has been achieved. The trance induction methods that follow are those which I use with my clients who attend to become non-smokers.

Evoking a memory of relaxation or creativity

The basic principle of effective hypnosis is explained by Milton Erickson in the following words:

> "[T]he hypnotized person remains the same person. Their behavior only is altered by the trance state, but even so, that altered behavior derives from the life experience of the patient and not from the therapist. At the most the therapist can influence only the manner of self-expression …
>
> "For example, anesthesia of the hand may be suggested directly, and a seemingly adequate response may be made. However, if the patient has not spontaneously interpreted the command to include a realization of the need for inner reorganization, that anesthesia will fail to meet clinical tests and will be a pseudo-anesthesia.
>
> "An effective anesthesia is better induced, for example, by initiating a train of mental activity within the patient himself by suggesting that he recall the feeling of numbness experienced after a local anesthetic, or after a leg or arm went to sleep, and then suggesting that he can now experience a similar feeling in his hand. By such an indirect suggestion the patient is enabled to go through those difficult inner processes of disorganizing, reorganizing, reassociating, and projecting of inner real experience to meet the requirements of the suggestion, and thus the induced anesthesia becomes a part of his experiential life instead of a simple, superficial response."[2]

In the same way as Erickson's example with anaesthesia, what we need to do with each stage of trance induction is to bring back the memory of the experience we want to invoke. When we want to bring about a fixation of attention on a single point, instead of using an external object such as a candle, crystal ball, swinging watch or hypno-disc, we focus the client's attention on an internal thought – a memory of a fascinating experience. When we want the client to feel relaxed, we invite them to recall a situation when they felt relaxed. When we want to bring about deepening, or dissociation, we talk in terms of the client's previous experiences of detachment from immediate surroundings. When we want to bring about the use of the client's creative imagination in order to bring about a solution, we encourage them to re-experience a previous successful use of that creative imagination. When we want to bring about smoking cessation, and the client has successfully stopped smoking in the past, we encourage the client to bring back that experience and repeat that success. If the client has not stopped smoking before, then we can bring back a memory of healthy and happy functioning as a non-smoker from the early years of life before they started smoking. This is the principle of utilisation: making use of existing resources from the client's repertoire of experiences in order to bring about the result we are seeking.

At the same time, it is essential to reiterate that the smoking issue is fundamentally different from those others with which hypnotherapists deal. The end result of the session must be that the client becomes a non-smoker, and therefore these Ericksonian techniques must be supplemented with plenty of direct and unambiguous suggestions to stop smoking and stay stopped.

"Day and Night" style of induction

To induce trance based on a memory of relaxation, first of all keep your ears open early in the session for any mention the client might make of pleasant and relaxing leisure activities that they enjoy, such as playing golf, gardening, yoga or playing a musical instrument. If there is such a leisure activity, then utilise that. If not, ask, "Have you been on holiday over the past year?" If the client replies, "Yes," then you ask, "Where did you go?" The client might say, "Cyprus."

THERAPIST: "Was there any particular day in Cyprus you particularly enjoyed?"

CLIENT: "Yes, just hanging out on the beach."

THERAPIST: "And what was that like, just hanging out on the beach?"

CLIENT: "Just totally comfortable. I felt free, able to completely unwind."

THERAPIST: "And I wonder if you can remember what that was like, being just totally comfortable – free – able to completely unwind?" (Pause.) "And can you remember the heat of the Mediterranean sun warming your skin? And could you hear the sound of the waves rolling onto the shore in an endless rhythm? And can you remember that more easily with your eyes open or *closed*? And could you see any other people there, just lying absolutely still and completely relaxed? And could you smell that smell of seaweed on the fresh air? While the heat of the sun spread through your skin down to the muscles beneath, warming those muscles, loosening them. So that all the areas of stress and tension just melted away as you became ever more comfortable, free and able to completely unwind." (If the client's eyes are not yet closed:) "So that your eyes can close any time they want to. And I wonder whether you found that your mind wandered freely, so that you could *lose track of time*, so that it didn't really matter whether you'd been there for seconds or minutes or hours or days. In fact, you could stay there for as long as you want – even as the sun begins to sink towards the horizon, and the sky turns orange and pink and purple, shadows get longer, a cool evening breeze blows from the sea, caressing your face and hair, the sound of the sea changes with the tide. And you could stay there even as the sun goes down and the vast night sky comes out – thousands of bright stars. And the moon rising and casting a pale white light over that scene …"

This is pacing and leading. We are bringing back both the client's description of their memories of that beach in Cyprus and aspects of that experience that almost certainly would be there, such as the heat, the sound of waves and other people lying relaxed and motionless on that same beach. Again, we hedge our bets by putting these memories forward in the form of questions or open-ended statements such as "Can you remember …?" and "I wonder whether you can recall …?" The purpose here is to overload the client's conscious mind with numerous items of information from a pleasant relaxed experience from their own memories, in which they entered a form of trance spontaneously. At the same time you put in subtle suggestions for eye closure. It is helpful, but not essential, to achieve eye closure to induce trance. The advantage of eye closure is that it blocks off the visual field so that the client's focus of attention, concentrated on internal experiences, is less likely to be distracted by something they can see. However, a perfectly adequate trance state is often achieved while the client's eyes remain open. In such cases, ensure that you remain as motionless as possible so as to avoid the risk of distracting the client.

In the final sentences, when you talk about sunset followed by night, you are now leading your client towards the hypnagogic state that you want them to experience. As day is replaced by dusk, then sunset and nightfall, people enter a different, more relaxed state which is more conducive to hypnosis anyway. This is particularly pronounced when we are in direct contact with nature, often on holiday. By leading the client in this way, we are simply bringing in the memory of what they have experienced every single night of their life.

Nor is it necessary that the client's memory of a holiday be a completely passive and relaxed one. If the client remembers an enjoyable day skiing, then you similarly feed back their experience and give a description of those aspects of the experience which were necessarily present. So you might say:

> "And I wonder if you can remember right at the start, standing on top of that piste, looking down at that vast expanse of whiteness stretching far, far down below. And breathing that thin, cold mountain air, while feeling those skis underneath your boots and the poles in your hand. And what was it like pushing down with that pole, so that you started to slide down that mountain? And just bending your knees to increase speed as you hear the howling of cold air in your ears and the wind-chill effect as that icy cold air blasts you in the face as you slide down, faster and faster down that mountainside. Those skis slicing through that snow as you found you could just tilt slightly left and right to steer yourself whatever direction you wanted to go. And I wonder whether you enjoyed doing a slalom around obstacles – whether you could leap through the air over a ridge and land softly on that snow below – enjoying that freedom of feeling – freedom of movement – losing track of time and space as you just experienced the moment in the moment …"

You then have the option of leading by describing dusk, the sunset, nightfall and moonrise as in the example above – if you think it is necessary.

Whatever holiday the client experienced, give as much detail as possible. Use all three modalities (visual, kinesthetic and auditory) with the descriptions you give to every client. Whilst for many individuals one of those modalities doubtless predominates, in practice everyone can operate in all three modalities to some extent – so use them all. The remaining two modalities – gustatory (G) and olfactory (O) can also be added where relevant. For example, if the client remembers a particularly delicious meal or trying out perfumes while shopping, then G and O will necessarily be significant modalities to which to refer.

Remember that holidays are not always a good experience. If the client tells you that the holiday was not pleasant, then pace that by saying, "I know. Often holidays can be more stressful than everyday life. I've had plenty of trips where I needed a holiday when I got back." Similarly, if they did not go on holiday over the past year, then you might ask, "Can you think of a situation, maybe in the past few months or maybe further back in the past, where you felt relaxed?" The client could describe a pleasant social occasion, or a visit to a spa, or simply taking it easy at home at the weekend. Whatever the client recalls, feed back their description of that experience to them, adding any elements that are likely to have been present, just as with the beach and skiing examples above.

Occasionally, the client may not want to give you any information about the memory they are recalling. I asked one male client to recall a relaxing experience. I said, "I wonder if you can remember what you were doing, what that was like?" He said, "Do I have to tell you?" I said (observing his non-verbal communications):

> "Of course not. You can just experience it right now, and as you remember what you could see and feel and hear, just letting that smile spread across your mouth will lead to those muscles becoming loose and limp and comfortable. And as your breathing is slowing and becoming deeper and more even, so you may notice just how pleasant and relaxing and comfortable that whole experience really was. That's right. Really experiencing that comfort now, so that maybe you can find that moment where you could completely lose track of time and enjoy purely that sensation … of well-being."

The nature of the experience he was recalling can be left to the imagination. The point is that you, the therapist, do not need to know any more than the client chooses to reveal.

Utilising the client's leisure activity to induce trance

As explained above, in the early stages of the session, you are constantly listening to the client's communications and making mental notes of resources that they already possess and refer to. It could be that the client mentions any number of experiences which you can utilise for trance induction, as with the holidays. You are particularly interested in those leisure activities which fascinate and absorb them, and which preferably also involve relaxation, creativity or both.

For instance, if the client has mentioned that they play golf, then ask,

> "I wonder if you can remember that round of golf in which you got your lowest ever score." (Pause.) "I wonder if you can remember what it was like standing at the first hole, taking out the driver, letting it swing for a moment as you built up your strength – teeing off, driving that ball down the fairway. Following it down, knocking it onto the green, just putting it with enough of a touch so that it rolled into that hole and no further. And can you recall how you felt as you got low score after low score and really began to realise that this was going to be one of your very best ever rounds?"

In the above, we are tapping into an experience of resourcefulness and a sense of personal achievement, as well as simply inducing trance.

Another example might be something musical, such as singing, composing or playing an instrument. Here you might say, "You play the guitar. And do you play your own compositions or other people's?"

> CLIENT: "My own."

> THERAPIST: "I wonder if you can remember a composition that you particularly enjoyed writing. And I wonder how that piece of music first came into your mind. Did it just start playing fully formed, might you have played a few chords and experimented, just to get a sense of harmony and melody and speed and mood? I wonder if you can remember that point where the music just took over and formed a life of its own, playing freely so that you could hear it in your own mind. That music taking form from your creative imagination. And isn't it interesting how music can take on a visual form in your own mind as you listen to it – and a feeling form so that you can sense it. As if that sound was also becoming swirls and shapes and flows of energy which you can see and feel as well as hear …"

In the above you are pacing from the auditory modality and leading to the visual and kinesthetic modalities. This "unity of the senses" is known as synaesthesia. This is an example of how you can add elements which you know to have an hypnotic effect in order to achieve trance ever more deeply. Naturally, the same principles apply, for instance, with a client who paints, or writes, or who engages in some craft such as making pottery, or renovating old clocks or car engines.

Adding colour to your descriptions strengthens the impact of the trance induction. A powerful way of inducing an hypnotic trance is to show the colours of the rainbow in succession: red, orange, yellow, green, blue, indigo, violet. It is unlikely that you will have lighting equipment capable of doing that in the therapy room, so you have to use words instead. In practice, indigo and violet are combined into a single colour – purple. Also, add the colour white to the end of that sequence, because in the context of lighting, white is a combination of all the colours. So the sequence is: red, orange, yellow, green, blue, purple, white. To achieve an hypnotic trance, rather than simply reciting the colours in order, put the sequence of colours into a context which has meaning and value for the client. So if the client mentions that they enjoy gardening as a pastime, then you can combine that interest with the use of the colours by assigning the colours to different flowers and plants. You might say:

> "And I wonder if you can remember a particularly pleasant day of gardening. Maybe one of those days in early spring when the weather is just starting to get warmer, and as you look at your garden, so you can see the bare brown empty flower-beds, the green lawn, maybe bare trees and bushes – and you can also see in your mind's eye the way that garden is going to be in the future – that mass of vibrant colour and life when all those plants and flowers have sprouted and grown into their mid-summer glory. So that already, as you're kneeling down in the spring, digging up that flower-bed with a trowel, tearing out the weeds, discarding pebbles, and planting those new seeds and bulbs, so too at the same time your creative imagination is already experiencing that beautiful garden of the future, in which you can see and smell those flowers and their petals, gently flowing in the breeze of summer, taking pleasure in the knowledge of how your skill and love has nurtured and grown them – perhaps the red of roses, the orange of sunflowers, the yellow of daffodils, the green of leaves and ferns, the blue of hyacinths and bluebells, the purple of heather and violets, the white of lilies and orchids …"

Here you are tapping into the client's creative imagination as well as inducing a doubly powerful trance by both overloading the client's conscious mind with sensory memories of gardening and using the colours in a relevant context.

The key strength of this method of trance induction is that the client remains firmly in their comfort zone. You are bringing back and utilising their positive memories of some activity that they enjoy. The key is to find and work with the client's enthusiasms, not yours. Find the activity, if any, that they really enjoy, love doing and enjoy talking about. Communicate in terms of that activity.

Needless to say, your own personal preferences are irrelevant. Although I have tried playing golf, I disliked it and was useless at playing it. But when my client is a golfer I talk about it as if I was just as enthusiastic as they are about it. That is because I am working, not the client. The therapist's task is to make the client's entire experience of the session as pleasant, comfortable, inspiring and results-oriented as possible. This is achieved by talking about the client's interests, not the therapist's. Of course, there are many things which you are enthusiastic about and really enjoy doing and discussing, but only use them for trance induction if it happens that a client mentions them as one of their own interests.

For clients who already practise some form of meditation, when you want to induce the main trance, utilise their particular method in order to do so. This means that you should be familiar with the different styles of meditation and be able to talk about them in a way which sounds to the client as if you know something about it. So whenever you come across a meditative technique previously unknown to you, look it up in a reference book or on the Internet and make a mental note of the basic concepts involved. If the client does mention a method which you are not familiar with, then you can say, "Excellent. Can you tell me something about that, and how you experience it?" You can then utilise and feed back the client's description as a means of enabling them to re-enter trance.

While it is undoubtedly useful for the lay hypnotherapist to have a general knowledge of the various meditation techniques, complementary and alternative therapies and so on, the point is that you do not need to have *much* knowledge about them. Make sure you understand the key concepts, and then, once you know some key words, you can effectively weave those words into your induction so that they trigger the client's memory of actual experiences. This helps rapport.

Yoga is increasingly popular and is likely to crop up most often. The following induction derives from yogic philosophy and practice, and is effective with anyone who has done any yoga at all:

> "You already know all about yoga. And I wonder if you can remember a really good yoga session that you have experienced. Can you recall sitting there in the lotus position perhaps, or maybe some other position, breathing in and out, in and out, in an endless rhythm. Focusing your attention on that moment between the breaths, while continuing that breathing in an endless flow. Because breathing is the beginning of life, an endless cycle of harmony with the energy and life of the universe. And every time you breathe out, be aware of the energy flowing through your body, mind and spirit.

"You already know that yoga means 'union' – the quest for an ultimate union of self with the universe. And these yoga exercises and meditations that you have already experienced are merely steps towards that ultimate union.

"The ancient yogic masters taught that there is a vital life energy, called *prana*, which flows through the universe and through the human body. Within the human body are seven different *chakras*, or energy centres, each associated with a specific colour, through which that prana flows. The word 'chakra' means wheel or disc or circular object. And as the prana flows upwards through the body, so each chakra is energised, and the wheel or circle spins round rapidly. The chakras are compared with drooping flowers, which raise themselves up like sunflowers facing the sun as the life energy flows upwards through them.

"The ancient masters taught that every human being is a tiny inlet of prana which is connected with the vast ocean of the prana in the universe, from which an infinite supply might be drawn. Let yourself breathe in that life energy from the universe, now.

"And be aware of that energy flowing through the first chakra, which is located at the base of the spine. The root chakra it is called. Be aware of the colour red, the colour of the root chakra. See red roses in a flower bed, a red carpet, the red of a pillar box, the red of a London bus, the red of the uniform of the Queen's guard. Fill your inner eye with the colour red as the prana energises the first chakra, at the base of the spine.

"Be aware now of the second chakra, located on the spinal column in the area of the reproductive organs. And as the energy rises to the second chakra, be aware of the colour orange. See a bowl of oranges, a jug of orange juice, the orange of a Buddhist monk's robe. Let your whole awareness be filled with the colour orange.

"And as the life energy rises through your body, it reaches the third chakra, located in the spinal column in the area of the solar plexus. See the colour yellow, the colour of the third chakra. See buttercups in a field, a bowl of daffodils, see the yellow sand of the desert, stretching to the horizon. Let the colour yellow fill your awareness as the energy flows through your solar plexus chakra.

"Be aware now of the colour green, the colour of the fourth chakra, the heart chakra, located in the spinal column in the area of the heart. See the green grass of a meadow, the green of leaves on a tree in summertime, the green of ferns, the green of an emerald. Fill your mind's eye with the colour green as the prana energises the heart chakra.

"And now, as the prana rises through your body, it reaches the fifth chakra, located in the area of the throat. Fill your inner awareness with the colour blue.

The blue of a cloudless sky in mid-summer, the blue of the ocean underneath the sky, the blue of a sapphire – see the colour blue as the energy flows through the throat chakra.

"And the sixth chakra is located in the pineal gland, in the forehead between the eyes, in what is known as the third eye. As the energy flows through the third eye, fill your awareness with the colour purple. A bowl of violets, a hillside covered with heather, the purple robe of a king. Let the colour purple fill your mind's eye as the prana energises the third eye chakra.

"The seventh and highest chakra is the crown chakra, located on top of the head, but extending above and around it like a bird hovering over its nest. As the life energy floods through the crown chakra, fill your awareness with the colour white. See the white of snow on a mountain top, the white of a polar bear's fur, the white of a lotus floating on a pond. For the crown chakra is known as the thousand-petalled lotus, a focus point for the white, warm energy of the universe. Be aware of that white, warm energy, flowing into and out of the crown chakra in a thousand rays of white light. Let that white light, that warm energy, spread now throughout all your seven chakras, throughout every part of you, energising, invigorating, transforming. Just experience it freely flowing through you.

"And as you experience this flow of harmony, this freedom of feeling, this attachment to the energy of the universe, so you gradually become aware that it's possible, perhaps inevitable, that you lose track of time. So that it doesn't matter if it's morning or noon or afternoon or evening or night. For time has no meaning in this transcendent state. And space, too. It doesn't matter whether you're inside or outside. In this wonderful exalted state you can travel freely through time and space, letting that prana, that life energy, transport you wherever you want to go ..."

Many people hold that the chakra model corresponds closely with their unconscious representation of the world. This induction will both get your clients into a deep trance and make sense to any who have experienced yoga or other Eastern-oriented meditative and spiritual practices.

The same of course also applies if the client tells you that they have enjoyed a relaxing experience during acupuncture, massage, reiki, aromatherapy or any kind of healing. Utilise the client's experience in the same way.

Present Experience Progressive Relaxation Induction

A minority of clients have difficulty recalling appropriate experiences. One of the following three things happens:

(1) the client struggles to access such a memory;
(2) the client cannot remember an experience of being relaxed;
(3) the client does not enter trance, and simply stays listening to the therapist's words with eyes open in full conscious waking awareness.

The moment it becomes obvious that one of these three situations is happening, pace the client by saying, "That's fine." If the client expresses any doubt about their ability to enter trance, or your ability to induce it, then you say, "Everyone's a unique individual. Everything you experience is authentic – there's no right or wrong in any of this. We'll find your individual way to become relaxed." Then you continue with what is called the Present Experience Progressive Relaxation Induction.

Most hypnotherapists are aware of the progressive relaxation induction. The concept of "progressive relaxation" was developed in the 1920s by Edmund Jacobson of Chicago University. In its original form it had no connection with hypnosis. The concept is that complete physical and mental relaxation can be achieved by first tensing, then relaxing, different muscle groups, working through the entire body until it is completely relaxed. In its original form, it is a long-drawn out process of conscious work in focusing, tensing and relaxing. Later researchers came up with quicker and simpler techniques for progressive relaxation than Jacobson's original version.

Later still, hypnotherapists adapted the concept of progressive relaxation as possibly the best known method of inducing trance. Essentially, it is an authoritarian technique, in which the hypnotherapist is telling the client what to do. Now there is a problem with authoritarian techniques. Time and again one meets people who have been for hypnotherapy who say, "I just sat there and didn't feel any different," or "I was just going along with it." If you simply tell a person to relax the different parts of their body by reciting a progressive relaxation induction script, then you cannot be sure that the client is in fact responding to the suggestions you are giving.

To avoid this problem, draw from the client a description of their *present* experience, and utilise and feed that back in the form of a progressive relaxation induction.

Induction

You ask the client, "How are you feeling right now?" The client is likely to give you a word, such as, "Comfortable." You ask, "And which part of you feels most comfortable?" The client might say, "My hands." You say,

"So I wonder if you can focus on those hands now. And just be aware of what precisely you can be aware of in those hands that tells you that those hands are comfortable. Notice the details of feeling that you can label with that word "comfortable". And is there anything you can see in those hands that you can identify as being comfortable? Is there some colour there that you can associate with being comfortable?"

The client might reply with a colour, such as, "Orange." So you continue,

"And as you become more aware of that comfortable feeling, and that colour orange in your hands, I wonder if you could spread that feeling and that orange colour up from your hands to your wrists, and then through your forearm up to your elbows, and then spreading that feeling of comfort and that orange colour up to your shoulders, so that the whole length of your arms becomes just as comfortable, just as relaxed, just as peaceful, as those hands are? And as you feel that comfortable sensation and that colour all the way up those arms, so you can let them spread across your shoulders, loosening all those shoulder muscles, and flowing up your neck, and around your scalp, melting all the areas of stress and tension as the muscles become more and more comfortable as that orange colour envelops them. So that that orange feeling of comfort can spread down your chest, descending and loosening and permeating all of those muscles. Down your back, relaxing all the muscles, large and small, inside and outside. Flowing through your stomach, down your hips, that comfortable orange spreading down your legs, all the way down to your feet, as that sensation descends down to the tips of your toes. So that your whole body is now just as comfortable, just as permeated with that orange sensation, as your hands …"

You are getting a description from the client of their present experience, asking how they feel in one particular part of the body, how they can identify that feeling, and then suggesting that the feeling spreads through one adjacent part of the body after another. This way you know that you are connecting with the client's actual immediate experience, and leading in the simplest possible way to the degree of bodily relaxation that you are seeking. You will get a satisfactory trance state with almost all clients using this technique.

Using instant self-hypnosis as a way to induce the main trance

There are still perhaps three to five percent of clients who are simply unable to tap into either past or present experiences that can be utilised for trance induction. In that case, once again, you validate the client. As soon as you realise that the client "just isn't getting" the Present Experience Progressive Relaxation Induction, you say, "That's fine. Do you remember the instant self-hypnosis we did earlier on?" Client: "Yes." Therapist: "How would you like to do that now?

Are you comfortable in that chair?" Client: "Yes." Then you simply repeat the instant self-hypnosis which you did earlier in the session, as described in the previous chapter.

As the instant self-hypnosis is repeated, visually check that the client has their eyes closed and is breathing correctly. The means that the client is at least in an hypnotic state which is satisfactory for the subsequent work of enabling them to become a non-smoker. The remaining two suggestions from instant self-hypnosis – saying the word "calm" silently and mentally, and seeing the word "calm" – are astoundingly simple. If the client can do one or both of them as well, then they will be in a satisfactory trance state to continue the session successfully.

Hypnotherapists will know the classic external features of trance. The breathing is slow, deep and even, the facial muscles become still, the face becomes paler, the pulse slows (this is visible at the neck, wrist and sometimes leg) and there can be slow and sluggish unconscious movements and often rapid eye movement. If you observe some or all of these, you know that trance is being achieved. If not, just continue as if you did observe them. Your message will still get through. Remember that the client is interested in becoming – and staying – a non-smoker. The client is not interested in whether particular hypnotic phenomena or depth of trance are achieved.

The learning set

For everyone, at some stage in the past, learning has moved from being conscious to being unconscious. You no longer have to think about what to do – you just do it. The function of the "learning set" in hypnotherapy is to describe to the client their previous experiences of unconscious learning by talking about the achievements they have attained in the past. In this way, you are both tapping into the client's faculty for unconscious learning and empowering the client by building up a self-image of creativity and resourcefulness. You talk about the things they have learned unconsciously as if they were the simplest and most natural things in the world – which of course they are, from the client's point of view. The purpose is to create the assumption that learning at an unconscious level to become and live as a non-smoker will be just as simple and natural. A straightforward approach to the learning set is the following:

"And ever since the day you were born, your unconscious mind has been helping you to learn, helping you to adapt successfully to new situations. When you first looked at the world, it seemed like a mass of undifferentiated shapes. But pretty soon your unconscious mind learned to judge the sizes and shapes and distances of different objects, so that you could easily navigate your environment.

"And when you learned to walk, can you remember how difficult that might have seemed? How you put one foot in front of the other, how maybe you kept stumbling and falling down, standing up again, until little by little you managed to find your balance, put one foot in front of the other, and pretty soon you could walk forward without even needing to think about it at a conscious level.

"And in the same way, you learned to run, to climb, and to do so many other things.

"And when you first learned to read, can you remember the first time you saw all those black shapes on that white paper? And how little by little, you learned the difference between those letters: the little *b* and the little *d*, the little *p* and the little *q*. Pretty soon, you learned the difference between the letters, and you went on to learn words and phrases and sentences, so that you could read a whole page of writing without even needing to think about it at a conscious level – that's because the unconscious part of your mind had learned how to read."

In the above passage, you have provided specific examples of unconscious learning from the client's early life. These are pacing statements: the client recognises them to be true. Your goal now is to lead the client towards accessing more general examples of unconscious learning from their life by using non-specific language. So continue:

"And later on, as you grew up, your unconscious mind enabled you to learn so much about life, about people, about yourself, in much the same way."

The purpose of the above passage is to elicit other examples of unconscious learning, in the areas of "life" in general, in social relations and in self-knowledge. You do not know what these examples are, but the client's unconscious does. Then your goal is to lead the client towards the idea of becoming a non-smoker through the same process of unconscious learning. Continue:

"And your unconscious mind is helping you to learn again today, [name], helping you to learn something of great benefit to you, your health and your future."

The above passage does not specifically mention the smoking issue. Instead, it refers to it indirectly ("something of great benefit to you, your health and your future"). Of course, the client knows that the purpose of the session is to quit smoking. The goal is to lead the client to the assumption that since they have already learned so many things unconsciously, it is reasonable and taken for granted that they can also learn to become a non-smoker.

In order to maximise the effectiveness of the learning set, it is a good idea to utilise skills and enthusiasms which you know the client already possesses. For instance, if the client has talked about traffic jams or the difficulty in finding a parking space, then you know that they drive a car. You might then say:

> "And can you remember when you first learned to drive, how there were so many things to think about? Clutch control, braking, accelerating, changing gear, indicating, looking in the rear view mirror, left turns, right turns, reversing, driving on the motorway, parking. Little bit by little bit, the more you practised, the easier it became, so that pretty soon you found that you could drive without even thinking about it at a conscious level. So that today, you can get behind the wheel of a car and you can be talking to a passenger or listening to the radio or thinking about what you're going to do when you get there, while your hands are steering the wheel, indicating, changing gear, your feet moving up and down on the brake and the accelerator, your eyes darting up to the rear view mirror – that's because the unconscious part of your mind has made you a master of driving."

You can make reasonable deductions about learnings that your clients have already attained simply by looking at them and listening to what they have to say. If the client walks into your consulting room carrying a crash helmet, heavy leather gloves and all the other paraphernalia, then it's reasonable to assume they have learned how to ride a motorcycle. So you simply adapt the above description of the learning set to the process of learning how to ride a motorbike. You might say:

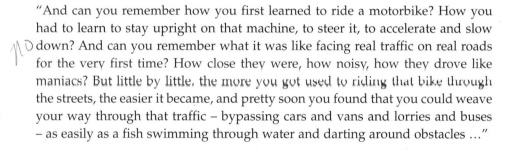

> "And can you remember how you first learned to ride a motorbike? How you had to learn to stay upright on that machine, to steer it, to accelerate and slow down? And can you remember what it was like facing real traffic on real roads for the very first time? How close they were, how noisy, how they drove like maniacs? But little by little, the more you got used to riding that bike through the streets, the easier it became, and pretty soon you found that you could weave your way through that traffic – bypassing cars and vans and lorries and buses – as easily as a fish swimming through water and darting around obstacles …"

In the same way, you can utilise other unconscious learnings which the client has achieved, by drawing on and describing the processes which are necessarily present in the shift from conscious to unconscious learning. If the client's mother tongue is not English, but they have learned English to a level of fluency, then you can say:

> "And can you remember when you first learned English? How many words you had to learn. And how quickly people seemed to speak in English. And how you kept translating in your mind between English and your native language, and your native language and English. Little by little, the more you learned, the more you listened, the more you spoke and read and wrote in English, the easier it became. So that the time came when you found that you could have

a conversation in English, watch TV in English, read a newspaper in English, even think in English – without needing to translate into your native language at all. That's because your unconscious mind made you a master of the English language."

If you know what your client's native language is, then substitute the specific language for the words "your native language" in the above passage. Equally, you can utilise any hobbies, interests or enthusiasms the client may have. The point here is to break down that process of learning into integral parts, giving as much detail as you may know about. For instance, if the client is a musician, you could say:

"And can you remember when you first learned to read music? Those lines on that page, with those little notes at different points on them? Learning the difference between the crotchets and the quavers and the semi-quavers and the rests. And the naturals and the sharps and the flats. And the difference between the various chords, learning melody and harmony and a sense of rhythm. And I wonder if you learned that with a metronome, moving back and forth, tick, tock, in an endless rhythm. Until the time came when you could just read a page of music and hear that composition just playing in your mind, without needing to think about the different notations on the page. That's because the unconscious part of your mind made you a master of the art of music. And in exactly the same way, your unconscious is helping you to learn again today, [client's name], helping you to learn something of great benefit to you, your health and your future."

The "forgetting set"

Next you talk about the learning set in the context of forgetting about interests which are no longer of value, moving forward towards an association with the process of abandoning the smoking habit. Just as the client's unconscious mind has already helped them to learn the skills and habits you have just mentioned, so too their unconscious has enabled them to forget many things that are no longer significant or relevant in present-day life. This is known as "the forgetting set".

You say:

"And just as your unconscious has found the way to help you learn in so many ways, so in exactly the same way, throughout the course of your life, your unconscious mind has left stuff back in the past which is no longer relevant to what's important to you now. When you were a very young boy/girl, you were probably very interested in toys and fairy stories and kids' cartoons and the tooth fairy. You probably enjoyed making sandcastles and eating jelly. Later on, when you became a teenager, you forgot all that young kids' stuff. As a teenager, you wanted to prove yourself, become part of the gang, come across as cool and glamorous and sophisticated. [If the client started smoking as a teenager, continue:] That teenage [name] focused on living in the moment. He/she was ready to try anything, to do anything. He/she had no knowledge of long-term health issues, or what was really important in life. And that habit of smoking started in the teenage years.

"Later on, you grew up, became an adult, and left the teenage way of doing things back in the past. As an adult, you learned to deal with people in a more grown-up, mature and responsible way. You took more responsibility, took a long-term view of what was important, built a career. [If you know it is relevant, you can add:] And when you got married, you took on responsibility for another person. And when you became a father/mother, you had to think about the interests of the whole family. In so many ways, you've left back in the past the teenage way of blowing tantrums, showing off, bunking off from things. Because that teenage [name] who took up that habit of smoking doesn't really exist any more, he/she's back in the past, and now as an adult, a grown-up, you're taking charge of your own life, your own health, and your own body, and you're not willing to risk that life, that health, that body for anyone, least of all that teenage kid who still had so much to learn about what's really important in life. As an adult, as a grown-up, you're choosing to take responsibility for your life, your health and your body, and you're going to leave back in the past that habit which that teenage [name] took up, back in the past where you left eating jelly and building sandcastles and all those other childhood and teenage things."

Of course, if the client started smoking as a young adult, instead of talking about teenage habits, you talk about young adult habits. You could say, depending on circumstances:

"As a young adult, moving to a new city with new friends/working with a whole bunch of smokers/living with a smoker, the younger [name] took up that habit of smoking in that temporary situation. But since then you've moved on in so many ways. You've found that you don't need to prove yourself to new friends/colleagues/your partner any more, and in so many ways you've matured, learned more and moved on. And in exactly the same way, today you're leaving back in the past that earlier habit which may have temporarily worked in that temporary situation, but today really doesn't do anything for you. Now that you know so much more about what's really important and worthwhile in life, you're taking charge of your health, your body and your life and you're not willing to risk them for anyone. Just as you've learned and moved on in so many other ways, so in the same way, you're leaving that temporary habit back in the past where it belongs …"

You are tailoring what you say to the client's unique situation, keeping the essential message clear.

Deepening

There are a number of metaphors employed for explaining hypnosis. The concept of "deepening" in hypnosis is widely used, but not universally so. Many academic studies have sought to classify hypnotic experiences into levels of "depth of trance" measured by "hypnotic scales". Various tests for different experiences (ideomotor responses, positive and negative hallucinations, anaesthesia, and so on) are regarded as signifying different levels on such a scale. This model sees hypnotic experiences as if they were a lift going down a mineshaft, descending to ever lower depths.

Another school of thought prefers to see awareness as a spotlight which can be shone in any desired direction in order to illuminate the required resources, whether internal or external, past, present or future, conscious or unconscious, real or imaginary. Within this model, dissociation occurs simply because the spotlight of awareness is being directed towards some internal experience rather than externally. You may find this metaphor more useful when the client is finding resources within themselves.

From a practical point of view, the concept of depth is a useful metaphor. It entails dissociation (that is, directing conscious attention inwards so that one can communicate with the unconscious without conscious interference), greater physical relaxation, and fulfilling the client's expectations (phrases such as "deeper and deeper" are well known to the public as being used in hypnosis).

The best-known method of deepening is counting either up or down. This draws on the innate human faculty of adding one plus one, which is the foundation of all mathematics, and which is an inherent faculty "hard-wired" into the human brain. Many hypnotherapists like to count down from ten to one (or zero). I prefer to count "down" from one to ten … and beyond, because that allows for going even deeper than the number announced – going down to twelve can be a surprise at the end of the count. By first telling the client that you are going to count down to ten, and then going beyond that to twelve, or twenty, the client is likely to follow along and go even "deeper" than they originally expected to go.

Another factor that adds to deepening is connecting the numbers to the hobby, interest or enthusiasm which we have already utilised to induce trance – or which otherwise has relevance to the client. For example, if the client has said that they enjoy cycling, and maybe you have used their description of a cycling holiday as a way of inducing trance, then you might say:

"And in just a few moments, I am going to count down from one to ten. And as I count down, so I'd like you to imagine that you are cycling down a country lane on the gentle slope of a hill in spring-time, from the hilltop down into the valley beneath. And as I count down from one to ten, so with each number maybe you can see by the side of the road ten road signs, with those numbers from one to ten. And as you pass each road sign, with each descending number between one and ten, your muscles are going to become one tenth more relaxed. Every number will take you ten percent deeper into this relaxed, comfortable and resourceful state. And if, as you descend down that hillside, past those road signs, you get a sense of sliding down freely, into your unconscious mind, into that part of you where real learning takes place, you can let that feeling take you all the way down. So ready, one, cycling down, two, down that hillside, three, a pleasant breeze in your face, four, and deeper and deeper, five, six, sliding down that hill under the power of gravity, seven, eight, drifting down, deeper and deeper, into the valley, nine, ten, (pause) eleven, and deeper and deeper still, twelve, and all the way deep down relaxed."

In the same way, if for instance the client enjoys cooking, you might say:

"And in a few moments, I am going to count down from one to ten. And as I do so, I'd like you to remember a meal you cooked that you particularly enjoyed making. And as I count down from one to ten, so too you can remember ten different ingredients for that meal – maybe vegetables you chopped up or herbs that you measured out or oil that you poured into a hot pan. And as you become aware of the sight and smell of each of those ten different ingredients with each descending number, so too your body will become ten percent more relaxed with each number and with each ingredient. Each descending number will take you one-tenth deeper into your creative imagination, into that part of you that remembers every experience and has always been there, helping you to learn and develop and move forward. So ready: one, two ..." (etc).

If when you observe the client, you judge that they need to go even deeper in order to achieve an adequate trance state, then continue in this way down to fifteen, twenty, or, exceptionally, thirty.

This method of deepening trance experiences using the concept of "descent" – as in skiing down a mountain or scuba diving – brings about a rapid and deep trance with dissociation. It seems that the unconscious part of the mind forms an automatic connection between the "going down" and "depth" of hypnotic trance on the one hand, and the physical process of descending from a mountain or into the undersea world on the other. You can also utilise the fact that some activities incorporate numbers as an integral part of what they are. For instance, there are 18 holes in a round of golf, so if your client is a golfer, then you would say something like,

"In a few moments in time, you will hear me count down from one to eighteen. And with each descending number between one and eighteen, so you can remember the best round of golf that you ever played. And with each number, so perhaps you can find your body becoming more and more relaxed, and your mind going deeper and deeper into that creative part of you where real learning takes place."

Connecting the process of hypnotic deepening to an actual experience of the client brings about greater relaxation and dissociation than just using numbers alone. Also, the client tends to forget any self-consciousness or misgivings about the process of hypnosis as they are doing – in imagination – something that they enjoy anyway, thereby staying firmly in their comfort zone.

Whatever interest or experience of the client that you use to deepen in this way, finish the deepening process with a suggestion for dissociation, as follows:

"So deeply relaxed, and in that part of you where real learning takes place, so you may find that your mind begins to wander – your conscious mind, that is – back to some pleasant memory, perhaps, or into your imagination, it doesn't really matter. Your conscious mind can go anywhere it wants – because it's the unconscious part of your mind that I want to speak to. And I want to speak to your unconscious mind about something of great significance – something significant to you, [name], to your health and your future …"

Talk about the dissociation in a breezy tone of voice, as if it's a trivial thing of no great importance, which is true enough, and then say the final sentence in an earnest and emphatic tone, as if it *is* a matter of great significance, which is also true.

The moment of decision

One purpose of inducing trance is essentially to eliminate the internal "noise" described by Kroger, so that the hypnotherapist's message reaches the client's unconscious without interference. At some point the client has made a conscious, deliberate decision to become a non-smoker. So now you want to validate and affirm that decision simply, directly and powerfully.

Trance is in part a process of physical relaxation of the muscles. Edmund Jacobson, the originator of progressive relaxation, recognised that, in a sense, we think with the muscles. Every time a person thinks about some experience or idea, there is always a certain tensing of the muscles in a certain configuration. If the muscles were completely relaxed, then there would be no conscious thought at all.

Now affirm the client's decision to become a non-smoker in the trance state. In the following passage, match the client's breathing by speaking when the client breathes out. You say,

"You have already decided to become a non-smoker. And because it is your choice to live as a healthy, happy non-smoker, that is why you stop smoking now and for the whole of your future life. It is your decision to become a non-smoker, [name], and you have, now, freed yourself from that smoking habit, forever and ever, because it is your choice to do so, and you can take pleasure in the fact that you are now a non-smoker."

Having affirmed that decision, continue by pacing the client's past experience and encourage their unconscious mind to enable their body to cleanse itself of the accumulated poison without experiencing cravings. You say:

"And when, as a teenager/young adult, you first took up that habit of smoking, maybe you can remember your body resisting. Perhaps you were coughing, feeling dizzy, wanting to be sick, even turning green. That's because your body was resisting that poison. The only way your body can communicate with you is through its bodily reactions, and when you were feeling sick, your body was saying, 'Stop it, [name]. That smoke is a poison, I don't want that smoke. Reject it. Stay a non-smoker.' But you forced your body to accept that smoking habit. And later on, when you wanted to quit smoking, maybe you found it difficult to quit, because your body didn't realise that you were quitting. But today, in this very relaxed state, in which your decision to become a non-smoker is becoming a reality, your unconscious mind now understands that you are now a non-smoker, and that fact, that understanding, can permeate every part of you, so that your body welcomes this breathing space that you are giving it, now that you are achieving freedom from the smoking habit."

Of course, if the client remembered taking up the smoking habit without any bodily symptoms of resistance, then omit the early description of the body resisting that habit.

Then, if the client has stopped smoking before for at least two weeks, you continue:

"And can you remember how good it was when you did stop smoking, for three whole months/two whole years [or however long the client stopped]? Can you remember waking up in the morning feeling fresh, breathing fresh, clean air into strong, clean and healthy lungs, with high energy flowing through mind and body? Can you remember looking in the mirror and seeing your skin fresh, young, healthy, energised? [Here you can add specific details which the client recalls, such as:] Can you remember how easy it was to run upstairs/work out at the gym/enjoyable it was to socialise/etc? Can you remember how good it was

119

to be able to live life, working, socialising, travelling, as a healthy, happy non-smoker? And enjoying that life for day after day, week after week, month after month and year after year [however long the client stopped for]? (Pause) I'd like to ask your unconscious mind to repeat that transformation now, so that once again you can enjoy that healthy way of life. Only this time you know all about self-hypnosis, how to create that relaxed, comfortable, resourceful state any time you want it, and how to be prepared for any and every situation, so that you stay a non-smoker in all situations. So this time you will remain a non-smoker for ever and ever."

In the event that the client has not stopped smoking for any length of time previously, you refer to their early life as a non-smoker, and specifically to the good day that you have already recalled and anchored:

"And can you remember how good it was for all those years of your early life when you lived as a healthy, happy non-smoker? As a young child, as a teenager, how you lived life and never once even thought about smoking? And can you remember that *one good day* during that non-smoking life that you experienced? I'd like to ask the unconscious part of your mind to bring back that experience now, so that once again you can live life as the non-smoker you were as a child and a young teenager. And now you know all about self-hypnosis, how to create that relaxed, comfortable, resourceful state any time you want it, and how to be prepared for any and every situation, so that you stay a non-smoker in all situations. So that you will remain a non-smoker for ever and ever."

Simplicity

Emphasise that it is a simple thing. Continue:

"So it really is that simple. You know that you're a non-smoker – so you don't smoke. You will never smoke tobacco again in any format. So that you don't smoke a cigarette or a cigar or a pipe or a roll-up containing tobacco. And if someone offers you a cigarette, all you have to say is, 'No thanks, I don't smoke,' and whenever you say that, your unconscious mind will welcome the fact that you are now a non-smoker. So you go through your daily life, and you find the whole focus of your attention shifting to the worthwhile, beneficial things all around you, focusing your thoughts on what's really important to you, so that you forget about that old habit. Smoking for you is the past, behind you. It all happened a long time ago. Just as you've moved forward, from being a young child, to being a teenager, to becoming an adult, (to becoming a husband/wife and father/mother [if these are relevant]), as you've left so much stuff back in the past as you've progressed, and changed the whole focus of your attention in so many areas to what's really important in life, so also you leave that old smoking habit in the past where it belongs, in the same place where you've left eating jelly and playing with toys and so much else."

Taking the client through a new day as a non-smoker

Then you describe to the client their typical day as a non-smoker. As you have made a mental note of what situations during the day they smoked in, you give a description of how it will be different – and preferable – to experience that same situation as a non-smoker. For instance, many clients will tell you that they "always" have a cigarette with their first cup of coffee in the morning, or when they want a break at work, or when they are out drinking with friends. So as you go through the client's day, make sure that you describe each situation differently, now that they are a non-smoker. You continue:

"And your unconscious mind can learn and recognise that you no longer want to smoke. So that you can take on board these suggestions, learn them just as you've already learned to walk, to run, to read, to write, to drive and so many other things that you have already learned to do at an unconscious level. So that you no longer have any desire to smoke when you awaken in the morning. And you can enjoy that taste of rich coffee in the morning so much better now that that film of tar has disappeared from the top of your tongue. And you have no wish to smoke when you stay in after breakfast, when you go outside. And while you are travelling – you simply do not want to smoke – whether you're travelling in a car, bus, train, boat, plane or simply walking – you simply do not want to smoke. And you have no desire to smoke while you are working. Now that you know all about ultradian rhythms and self-hypnosis, you can move yourself up and down that numerical scale to find just the right level of alertness and relaxation for every working situation. And as a non-smoker, your concentration improves, your reflexes get faster and energy level rises, so that you will achieve more and easier and better in your career, now that you are a non-smoker. You have no desire for tobacco after lunch or dinner, and by eating like a gourmet, giving your body the water-rich foods it really needs, you will become/remain just as slim as you want to be. And when you are partying, socialising, drinking and dining, you have no desire to smoke – whether it be with friends, family, colleagues, clients, people you know well or people you've only just met. [If the client mentioned stress as an issue:] You can bring yourself down to 20 on that numerical scale of alertness and relaxation just by practising that simple self-hypnosis. And you can trust your body to protect you from other people's poisonous smoke. And if anyone offers you a cigarette, you simply say, "No thanks, I don't smoke." You simply let the conversation move on, and pretty soon you forget about that moment.

"And it's as easy as that. You go through day-to-day life and find yourself focusing on what's really important to you – so that bit by bit you forget that you ever smoked. Smoking for you is in the past – only a memory – a slowly disappearing memory." [Here you mark this phrase by speaking more and more quietly as you pronounce those words.] "And maybe, as someone who used to smoke sometime back in the past, perhaps a stray thought, or mental picture about smoking might pass through your mind for a moment, and as a non-smoker you can simply let it pass through like so many other stray, random thoughts. No point in struggling with that stray thought – your mind will rapidly focus again on something more useful and valuable – so you forget about the whole thing, certain that you will always be a non-smoker."

Stressing the client's descriptions of the benefits

At this point refer back to the form the client filled in at the start of the session, in which they described the three main benefits gained from becoming a non-smoker. You can say:

"Indeed, insofar as your thoughts wander towards the whole area of this transformation you've brought about within yourself, you think of how much your life has improved now that you are a non-smoker." [Here you can intermingle what the client has written down with other benefits that you can think of.] "Thinking about how good it is to wake up in the morning, feeling fresh, breathing fresh, clean air into strong, clean and healthy lungs – with high energy flowing through mind and body. You think about how good it is to enjoy much better health, to know that you've greatly extended your life, greatly improved your long-term health prospects. Looking in the mirror and seeing your skin fresh, young, healthy, energised, your teeth clean and white and shiny. How good it is to have your senses of smell and taste come back to their proper level, so that you can enjoy the fresh, clean smell on your fingers, in your hair, on your clothes, in your home. Thinking about all the extra money that is now yours, and the worthwhile beneficial things you can spend that extra money on, things that will improve the quality of your life. Thinking about the social freedoms you now enjoy, how you can now go anywhere you like, do anything you want, and enjoy that experience. How happy those people are who mean so much to you now that you've made this transformation to excellent health and long life. You think of the excellent example you're setting to those whom you influence." [If the client is a parent, then:] "Did you know that your child(ren) is/are far more likely to grow up as (a) non-smoker(s) now that you are yourself a non-smoker? And you think of that sense of independence, knowing that you are free, [name], moving forward to a healthy future life of freedom."

Note that these benefits are couched in purely positive terms. There is no mention of illnesses or other unpleasantness associated with smoking. Your whole tone of voice and manner must convey a sense of reality and enthusiasm to the client as you discuss these benefits.

Ego-strengthening

The concept of "ego-strengthening" as a feature of hypnotherapy is associated with John Hartland, who used it with all of his hypnosis patients. Hartland claimed that the use of ego-strengthening increased success rates by up to 70 percent, compared with hypnotherapy without it.[3] The purpose of ego-strengthening is to build up within your client a high sense of self-esteem, capability and empowerment. As with all aspects of hypnotic communications, you can add in elements drawn from your client's unique experience and tailored to their needs. You could say:

"And day by day, week by week, month by month, as you become more and more used to life as a non-smoker, so your mind will become more and more clear and calm, while your body becomes more and more supple and relaxed. Finding your energy level rising as all that trapped physical and mental energy comes back at your disposal. So that you find it easier to live life resourcefully – drawing on the power you already possess within yourself to deal more effectively with the world, with the people you deal with, with every situation. Cultivating the habit of self-hypnosis, finding the most appropriate level of alertness and relaxation for every situation. Finding yourself enjoying life more, taking life in your stride, opening yourself up to those things that the unconscious really wants for you deep down. And as you leave that old unwanted habit back in the past where it belongs, so you find yourself positively embracing this better and healthier future."

You continue talking with that positive, enthusiastic tone of voice that you already used when talking about the benefits of becoming a non-smoker.

Future pacing and unconscious learning

Next, bring back the client's representation of the future date (a month or a year in the future) that you suggested earlier, when you taught the client self-hypnosis. If that representation was both clear and positive (in other words, the client saw themselves as a non-smoker on that future day), then you have a strong resource that you can utilise in future pacing and unconscious learning. Even if that was not the case, you still use whatever representation the client has of that future date, as it may have changed by now. You say:

"And I'd like you to take down now that photo album which shows [name's] future life. And have a look at the photo of [name] on 17th June 2010 [or whatever date was specified during the teaching of self-hypnosis earlier]. Notice the expression on his/her face, the way he/she holds his/her body, hear the things he/she is saying, and the things he/she can hear, and really notice the difference. And if you like what you can see and hear, then step inside [name's] body, so that you can feel the way your body feels, see the things you can see, and hear what you can hear, and really notice the difference. And I'd like to ask your unconscious mind to take just three silent minutes to find the best, the most powerful way to make this future a reality in your life. Three silent minutes to reflect on everything you've experienced, everything I've said, three silent minutes to make it happen. So just take three minutes to do that, starting now."

You then remain silent for three minutes, allowing the client's unconscious mind to develop the way to live as a non-smoker. This is probably the most powerful section of the entire session, as the work is taking place entirely within the client.

At the end of the three minutes, you wrap it up by saying: "And this process of learning, understanding and transformation can continue today, tonight, tomorrow and in the days ahead." This "benediction" encourages the work of transformation to continue at an unconscious level even after the client awakes to full conscious awareness.

The Milton model

Richard Bandler and John Grinder coined the term "Milton model" to describe the non-specific language patterns used by Milton Erickson in his hypnotherapy. Erickson used deliberately vague language in order to encourage the process of unconscious learning and transformation within his client. Erickson did not know exactly what was going on inside the client's unconscious, so he used phrases which had no content in themselves, but which the client's unconscious could find specific meanings for. An example of Milton model language is:

> "I know that you are wondering ... and it is a good thing to wonder ... because ... that means ... you are learning many things .... And all the things ... all the things ... that you can learn ... can bring you new insights ... and new understandings. ... And you can, can you not?"

These words are "content free" – they say nothing specific, but the client's unconscious mind can "attach" content to them in its own internal process of transformation. When you say the phrases above ("I know that you are wondering ..."), and do so with intensity and conviction in your tone of voice, with belief and passion that the client is achieving something dramatic, the client will respond appropriately at an unconscious level.

By this late stage in the session, assuming that the therapist's communications have been effective, a shift of internal resources has already started to take place within the client's unconscious mind. The purpose of using Milton model language is to pace the client, strengthen this unconscious process and lead the client towards becoming a non-smoker in their own way. As you cannot know exactly what is happening in this process, you simply speak vaguely but intensely in order to pace the client's internal experience and lead towards an effective outcome. Sometimes you might want to have a lighter, 'wondering', musing tonality.

It is as if you were to stand on a mountain-top and kick a small pebble, which falls onto a larger stone and dislodges it, causing it to hit a rock below, which in turn drops onto a boulder, thus setting off an avalanche. When you kicked that one tiny pebble, you could not predict exactly which stones would hit which rocks as a result, but you still caused an avalanche.

It is much the same with the use of the Milton model. You do not know exactly the effect that your words will have on the client's unconscious, but those words can still have the effect of causing the internal avalanche which turns a smoker into a non-smoker.

Awakening

It is best to awaken the client quickly, as this means that they will still be in a highly receptive state immediately after arousal from trance, which you can utilise. In order to awaken, you say:

> "So now that your unconscious mind has learned how to carry out this wonderful transformation in your life, I'm going to wake you. I will count from twelve to one [or whatever number you used in deepening], and you will wake up just a little bit with each number. Until on the count of three, your eyes will open, and by the count of one you will be completely awake. Every part of you will be back in the here and now, except that part of you that used to smoke, and you will awaken feeling great, optimistic, alert and energised, with a sense of achievement flowing through every part of you. So ready: twelve, eleven, ten, nine, waking up, eight, seven, six, coming back to the here and now, five, four, three, opening your eyes, two, one, wide awake, wide awake."

Allow the client time to come back to full waking awareness. In the event that the client does not awaken, you pace and lead by saying,

> "And the wonderful thing about unconscious learning is that it can continue even after you awaken and return to the here and now. So in a moment you will hear me count from five to one and you will wake up more and more with each number, until on the count of three your eyes will open and by the count of one you will be fully wide awake. So ready: five – waking up – four – waking up – three – opening your eyes – *opening your eyes – open your eyes*" (keep on until

either the eyes open or it is obvious that no matter how often you repeat that suggestion the eyes will not open) "two – one – wide awake, wide awake."

If the client is still in trance with eyes closed, then you can say, "And in a moment I'm going to blow gently on your eyelids. And when I do that, your eyes can open and you can return to full waking awareness. So ready …" Then you blow gently on the client's eyes. The client will awaken at this point.

After awakening

Once the client is back in full waking awareness, your first task is to focus attention on their present experience, and away from what they have just experienced in trance. You want to allow the client's unconscious mind to continue the work of transformation, free from interference by the conscious part of the mind.

Ask: "How are you feeling now?" with a slight emphasis on the word "now". The client will give you a description. Provided that it is a neutral or pleasant description (and it usually will be), you say, "Excellent. Anything else on your mind that you want to mention?"

The purpose of asking this question is to check your work. You need to find out, as far as it is feasible to do so, that the client has achieved what both of you set out to achieve during the session. You deliberately phrase this question in this way. It allows the client to mention something that was on their mind earlier on, or which is on their mind in the present moment. Also, it protects the client's privacy by encouraging them to say only what they want to mention. If the client says, "No" in response to that question, then you move on to the closure of the session.

However, a small minority of clients will say something like, "I still feel as if I could walk out of here and light up a cigarette." In that case, you ask, "How do you know that?" What you are doing is searching for the internal representation which tells the client that they want a cigarette. The goal is to change it rapidly and easily, using submodalities and affirmations. Because the client has just woken out of trance, they are still in a very receptive state in which there is a minimum of the internal noise which can often interfere with the work of change.

In answer to your question, the client might say, "I can just see myself walking out of here and lighting up the moment I reach the street." You then reply,

> "Have a look at that picture now. Can you shrink it down so that it's really small, the size of a postage stamp? And can you make it black-and-white, a still picture,

darken it, blur it? And can you move that small picture to the other side of your head? And that spot where that picture of you smoking was just a moment ago – in that same spot, I'd like you to place that picture of yourself as a healthy, happy non-smoker that you saw earlier on, when we were doing that self-hypnosis. And I'd like you to make that new picture big, life-size, in full colour, a moving picture. And if there's some piece of music that you find inspiring, then play that music as an accompaniment to that picture. And then step inside your own body in that picture and feel the way your body feels, see what you can see, and hear what you can hear. And say this affirmation to yourself: 'It's great to be a happy, healthy non-smoker. It's great to be a happy, healthy non-smoker.' Say that to yourself again and again, silently and mentally, in a confident, reassuring tone. 'It's great to be a happy, healthy non-smoker'." (Pause) "And how are you feeling now?"

In all likelihood, the client will tell you that they feel better and more optimistic. Then you say, "You see how easy it is to change what you can see and make it work for you rather than against you?"

Alternatively, when you ask for a description of how the client knows that they want to smoke, the client might say something like, "I can feel the smoke coming down through my lungs into this black mass in my stomach." Then you say,

"Can you focus on that smoke going down into your lungs now? And can you reverse the direction of that smoke, so that it's going up from that black mass in the stomach – up through the lungs and out of your mouth, like a film being shown in reverse? And can you imagine getting a can of spray-paint in a light, bright colour, and painting that mass in that light, bright colour? And can you shrink that light, bright-coloured mass until it's very small indeed, the size of a table tennis ball, and can you raise it up so that it reaches your forehead, while the smoke continues to flow upwards in reverse?"

Probably, the client will be able to make these simple changes and identify a recognisably improved representation. Again, you say,

"You see how easy it is to change how you feel inside and make it work for you instead of against you? And if at any point in the future you found yourself feeling that same sensation, you could reverse the direction of that smoke and change that mass in the stomach in exactly the same way, and you will be able to transform your experience just as you have here and now."

Having shown the client how to change the submodalities of their experience, you can then trigger the anchor which has previously been established during the teaching of self-hypnosis of memory of life as a non-smoker. You say, "Let's just do this." Then you press the client's wrist at the place previously anchored and say, "healthy"/"free"/"happy" or whatever the word was that was used. Repeat the word several times.

Then continue:

> "And say this affirmation to yourself again and again, silently and mentally: 'It's great to be a healthy, happy non-smoker. It's great to be a healthy, happy non-smoker.'"

Pause for a moment to let the client repeat that affirmation internally three or four times. Then say,

> "And if there's any piece of music that you find inspiring, then maybe you can hear that music playing in the background as you repeat that phrase in your mind again and again."

Pause to let the client "hear" the internal music while repeating the affirmation internally. Then ask: "What are you aware of now?" The client will probably tell you that they are experiencing a change of state in a positive direction now that the anchor is being triggered and the affirmation repeated. If so, you then say:

> "You see how easy it is to make an improvement in the way you feel? What we did then, with pressing those points on the wrist, was trigger an anchor. It's simply a way of bringing back a resourceful state that we need right now. Maybe you've had the experience of smelling a particular perfume or aftershave, which you haven't smelt for a long time, but when you do smell it, it brings back powerful memories of a particular person, and places and situations from the time when you knew that person. You can see them and hear them vividly. All we're doing by triggering this anchor is the same thing, by bringing back your experience of life as a healthy, happy non-smoker. And you can do that yourself any time you want in order to ensure that you stay a non-smoker."

A few clients, even at this stage, will express doubts or scepticism. Some will be unable to make the changes to their internal representations that you have endeavoured to achieve. A handful will still say that they are likely to smoke on leaving the premises. In such cases, your last resort is to say:

> "The future hasn't happened yet. If you commit to practising self-hypnosis, you can create calmness, relaxation and a peaceful state any time you want. And remember, it only takes two weeks for the body to clear itself out and become a non-smoker's body. The very worst that anyone experiences during that process of cleansing is physical cravings. Those cravings only last ten seconds. And if you can distract your mind for ten seconds, then they disappear. And remember, nobody has ever died as a result of giving their body that two weeks' breathing space to become a non-smoker. The simple fact is that throughout your life

you've committed to learning things where you can see the benefits of doing so. When you first learned to drive a car, you assumed that you could and would master all the different aspects of driving – and because you assumed that, it became both possible and easy. So what would happen now if you simply assumed that you could become a non-smoker, and learn to live in that healthy way just as easily as you've learned to drive?"

Fortunately, only a handful of clients will be unable (or unwilling) to change their representations, so only rarely will you have to give this last piece of advice. But a central point is that you, as the hypnotherapist, must be completely resolute and certain in the client's ability to become and stay a non-smoker, and unconditionally committed to their success – no matter what their attitude may be at any point. Unfortunately, a few clients will simply abandon the whole endeavour of becoming a non-smoker at some point or other and resign themselves to permanent smoking – but it must always be the client who "gives up" in this way, never the therapist.

It is essential you check your work and deal with whatever the client comes up with. However, the large majority of clients will affirm that they are okay and that everything is fine. So you continue:

> "The thing to do now is to focus on the positive, because we get more of what we think about. Remember, we're both here for one reason, to make this successful and to deal with your experience, so if at any time you feel that you'd benefit by coming back for a reinforcement session, you are most welcome to do so. It doesn't matter if it's a month from now, a year from now, it's included in the price." (Handing over your card.) "You might like to give me a call in a few days to let me know how you're getting on. What I'd like to do now is give you two CDs."

At this point you hand the client a CD containing a recording of your voice giving a self-hypnosis message to stay a non-smoker. You say,

> "This is the sound of my voice, giving suggestions for relaxation and to reinforce what we've done today. Don't know how much of that you want to hear after this morning/afternoon/evening." [The idea of this line is to get a laugh.] "If you remember the self-hypnosis we did earlier, you might like to listen to it whenever you do that. You could just keep it in the drawer for listening to any time you feel you'd benefit from hearing it."

Chapter 8

A self-hypnosis CD for your clients

There are three reasons for giving your client a self-hypnosis CD to take home and play. First, it enables the client to create a peaceful, calm, comfortable state any time they feel it would be beneficial. Second, it enables the client to continue the work after the session and deal with any experiences that come up. Third, an object given to the client becomes a symbol of healing which of itself enhances the prestige of the whole hypnotherapy process in the client's eyes and therefore makes it more effective.

Record the message on the CD in your own voice. You can either record it on your home computer or else, for best results, use a professional recording studio. You can make any number of copies of your master CD. You can duplicate a small number one-by-one on the CD re-writer on your personal computer. However, given that you are likely to be seeing at least hundreds of smoking cessation clients in your career, it is easier to order a batch of fifty or more from a company with machines designed for mass duplication.

The message on the CD should cover the main points you made during the first session. It should also prepare the client for successfully dealing with the situations likely to be faced in adapting to the non-smoking life. With the live one-to-one therapy you do with the actual individual client, you respond to the communications they give you. With the CD, by contrast, you are creating a generic, "one size fits all" message which has to cover all clients and the situations they are likely to face. The self-hypnosis CD should ideally be around fifteen to twenty minutes, and definitely no longer than 30 minutes. A script you can use which draws on the approach in the initial session – and which perhaps you can adapt to your own therapeutic style – is as follows:

> "All right, now make yourself comfortable. And with your *eyes closed*, I'd like you to be aware of your breathing. Breathe slowly, deeply and evenly, building up a nice, natural rhythm of deep, easy breathing." [Verbally mark these words by speaking slowly.] "That's right. And the best place to breathe from is your diaphragm, just below your lungs, where your abdomen is, as you already know. And as you're breathing from the diaphragm, so your stomach is going up and down, and that's just fine, because it means that oxygen is flowing to every part of the body, which is exactly what the body needs. Good. And every time you breathe out, can you expel all the air from your lungs, breathing in completely new air, so that you're getting a really good air circulation. That's right. And every time you breathe out, in your own mind, say the word "calm" to yourself,

silently and mentally. And every time you breathe out, see the word "calm", written right in front of you, written in your mind's eye. Good. And every time you do this, you'll be putting yourself into a peaceful, calm, comfortable state.

"And did you know that it's possible to let yourself become very much calmer and more relaxed than you are now? To let your body find its own level of comfort and peacefulness, tranquillity and ease. And your mind, too, for the mind and body are one system.

"And just be aware that throughout the course of your life you have achieved and learned and grown and moved forward. And your unconscious mind has been helping you to survive and thrive in one situation after another. As you have moved through life and gained an increasing sense of your own worth, your creative imagination has been helping you learn about life, about people and about yourself.

"So just imagine on the crown of your head a lump of the sweetest, most fragrant, coolest elixir – a lump the size of an egg. Let that cool elixir melt gradually downward through your skull into the brain, and down through the body beneath, filling every pore, flushing out all worries and cravings and tension as it spreads through the body, cooling the muscles, bones, bloodstream as it draws out the hot debris of stress and wear and tear and conflict, descending down the throat, through the chest, through all the muscles, down the arms towards the fingertips, down through the stomach, down the hips, down the legs, all the way down to the soles of the feet and toes. And as the warm elixir circulates back up through the body, the internal organs are purified, the skin becomes radiant, and the balance of body and mind is restored.

"And with this balance restored, you can detach yourself from the flow of conscious thoughts, that running commentary which runs continuously through your mind.

"That flow of thoughts can become like the reflections on the surface of a stream, flowing ever forward. So that you can become a witness to your thoughts flowing on the surface of that stream. Those thoughts which are useful and consistent with your present and future life as a healthy, happy non-smoker, and those other thoughts which are less useful and less consistent with your health – those cravings, stressful moments, maybe other thoughts that you have been unhappy with recently. So just take a few moments to lie there idly on the banks of that stream, observing that flow of thoughts drifting past on that surface – a witness to your thoughts. And you know that you could stay here looking at those thoughts for as long as you like. Losing track of time, just as you might lose track of time lolling by the banks of any stream on a warm pleasant day.

"And be aware that those thoughts that you can see flowing on that surface are all *your* thoughts – yours to choose from, yours to alter, yours to make effective for your health, your energy, your long life, your increased financial prosperity, your freedom. Just notice as one of those less useful thoughts starts to float by – maybe a craving, a temptation, a stressful thought – a thought you want to get rid of. And right next to you on the bank of that stream is a pile of heavy stones. And as that thought passes, pick up one of those stones, feeling its weight in your hand, and drop the stone into that stream, so that as that stone hits the water with a splash, it disrupts the surface, breaking up the pattern of that unwanted, undesirable thought, forming concentric circles which spread out to touch the banks of the stream. And really notice the difference. And then wait for the next such unwanted thought to come by, and drop in a second stone – splash! – into the water – so that the ripples from that stone break up the pattern of that unwanted thought. And now do that a third time – when the next unwanted thought passes, just drop that stone onto it, breaking it up and disrupting it. Letting the good and desirable thoughts pass through complete and intact.

"You see how easy it is to choose those thoughts which are consistent with your good health, long life, energy, prosperity and freedom? So just gaze at those good and positive and healthy thoughts on the surface of that stream now. Isn't it good to focus on those happy and positive and reassuring thoughts for a change? And just imagine the sun shining even more brightly on that surface, so that you can see them more brightly, in richer colour, in sharper focus.

"Look at the images of yourself living this healthy, happy life as a non-smoker. Waking up in the morning feeling fresh, breathing fresh clean air into strong, clean, healthy lungs. Feeling high energy flowing through mind and body. Your skin fresh, young, healthy, energised. Observe scenes from your new daily life – how different your daily routine is now that you've made this wonderful transformation. And any time you like, you can step into your own body in that image of your new non-smoking life, merge yourself with it, actually see it and hear it and feel it. Actually live this non-smoking life – and really notice the difference. (Short pause.) So you can recognise that your unconscious mind is making your choice – your decision – your commitment – to live as a healthy, happy non-smoker into a reality in day-to-day life.

"So that you simply do not want to smoke. You never touch tobacco again in any form ever again. You never smoke a cigarette or a cigar or a pipe or a roll-up containing tobacco. And if anyone offers you a cigarette or asks if you smoke, you will simply say, "No thanks, I don't smoke" and each time you say that this will confirm that you are a healthy, happy non-smoker.

"So that when you wake up in the morning, breathing easily and freely, there is no inclination to smoke – and getting ready in the morning, no taste for smoking – and when you are travelling, whether it be by car, train, boat, bus, plane or walking – no wish to smoke. And during the day, you have simply forgotten that old habit. And you can work with your ultradian rhythms, creating this sense of calmness and resourcefulness that you're experiencing right now, any time you want it. And you'll find your concentration improves, your energy level rises, your reflexes get faster – so you'll be able to achieve more and easier and better in your daily routine, now that you are a non-smoker. And after breakfast, lunch, dinner – you simply don't want to smoke. And by eating water-rich foods, really focusing on that food, eating small morsels and really enjoying that like a gourmet, you'll be able to stay just the weight you want to stay. And when you are socialising with friends, family, colleagues, people you know well or people you've only just met – there is no desire to smoke. And it doesn't matter if other people happen to be lighting up. They're living their individual lives and you're living yours. So the fact that they happen to be stuck in that habit means nothing to you. You can trust your body's natural defence mechanisms to protect you from the poison of other people's smoke.

"And it really is that simple. You go through daily life and forget about that old habit. It all happened a long time ago – it's all in the past – a slowly fading memory. While you find the whole focus of your attention shifting increasingly towards those positive, desirable things which are most important to you – those values and goals and achievements which you do want – opening yourself up to those things that your unconscious mind really wants for you, deep down.

"So you can find yourself now back on the bank of that stream, casually observing that flow of thoughts on the surface of the water. And when you know that those thoughts are fully consistent with your new life as a healthy, happy non-smoker, you can come back to the here and now, becoming awake and alert and refreshed, and allow your eyes to open."

In addition to the above, you might choose to give your clients a second CD for relaxation. Depending on your preference, this could contain New Age music, whales singing, the sound of a forest or synthesised sounds. My own choice is Baroque music from the years 1700 to 1750, when such music was composed in its purest form. I give my clients a CD entitled *Baroque music for self-hypnosis* (See Appendix 4 for details) which is a surprise gift which has not been announced in advance. I continue:

"And here's some Baroque music we've had specially produced. Baroque music is very useful for self-hypnosis, or for creating relaxation. It produces alpha waves within the brain, which are associated with relaxation, learning, meditation and self-hypnosis. So you might like to play it when you're doing self-hypnosis or else relaxing at home or even during the day, if that's possible. Baroque music is also associated with the healthy functioning of the body. The rhythm of Baroque music is 72 beats per minute, which is the same as that of the healthy human heart. As the mind and body respond to whatever sounds are in their environment, you may as well give them those sounds which are compatible with good health."

This extra CD is not only for the stated purpose, but also to induce in the client a good feeling about being given something unexpected.

Written handout

In addition to the self-hypnosis CD and the music CD, give the client a written handout containing details of simple but effective ways to be prepared for, and deal with, every situation in daily life once they have left your premises (an example is included on the accompanying CD-Rom). This handout enables the client to refer to the techniques easily and put them into practice in everyday life. Most clients will forget the techniques you have taught them orally during the session. If the techniques relating to instant self-hypnosis, stress management, focusing attention, staying slim and so on, are written down, then the client has them permanently available when needed.

Keep the presentation of the handout simple. Print on A4 sheets using a laser printer. The cover should be a simple plastic report binder with a transparent front (purchased from a stationery store). The client is more likely to keep a document presented in such a plastic cover than one which is either stapled or not bound at all.

As you hand over the document, you can say, "Here's a handout which describes the different techniques for making sure that you are prepared for every possible situation. It shows how to practise instant self-hypnosis, manage stress, stay slim, focus your attention and so on. [Of course, you can emphasise those issues of special concern to the individual client.] You might like to read through it and find those techniques which are useful in your particular situation, and work with them to help you adapt. Well, that's about it for today."

Then once the client has got up, you ask, "How would you prefer to settle up?" Then the client gives their preferred method of payment and you collect your fee. Ensure that the collection of the fee is smooth, quick and easy. Make sure that you have a functioning pen for payment by cheque and plentiful change for payment with cash. If you accept payment by debit and credit card, ensure your machine is functioning, and that you know how to use it. As you show the client to the door, you say, "Remember, feel free to call or e-mail me any time anything's on your mind. That's what we're here for."

Chapter 9

The follow-up session

On the phone: reframe relapse as a blip on the road to success

At the heart of the process of unconscious transformation lies a mystery. The precise internal mechanism which enables a person in hypnotic trance to experience the epiphany which turns them into a non-smoker is unknown. The hypnotherapist's task is to lead the client to that state where such an epiphany can take place, and to ensure that the client consciously knows how to stay a non-smoker afterwards.

Although some clients will happily become non-smokers for the rest of their lives, others will need a follow-up session. In general, most people are lazy when it comes to practising the self-hypnosis exercises you have taught them. Therefore I recommend that you offer a further session as a follow-up. If the client reverted to smoking after the first session, your task is to examine their experience and work to achieve success this time. If the client has stopped smoking but still wants a follow-up, your task is to help them adjust more easily to life as a non-smoker.

After the main smoking cessation hypnotherapy session, the client is likely to face such situations as a stressful day at work, an argument with a family member, going out drinking with group of friends who are all smoking (and, perhaps tempting the client with cigarettes in a "joking" manner), or taking a puff from a joint (containing both tobacco and marijuana) which is being handed round at a party. In other cases, clients will find dealing with the physical cravings very difficult and may succumb to them. Although you have done your best to prepare the client for such situations, the "hypnosis" manifested by the immediate situation can in many cases in the heat of the moment override what you did in the session. You have to make sure that your magic is more powerful than the magic created in those situations.

When the client calls you requesting a follow-up session, your first task is to reassure them that they can and will become and stay a non-smoker. Explain that the relapse was merely a temporary blip which they can learn from in order to achieve the success they desire. If the client has not yet relapsed, but is merely looking for help in adjusting to life as a non-smoker, say, "Excellent. When you come round, we'll work on ways of enabling you to adjust to life as a non-smoker, now that you're giving your body this breathing space. When would it be most convenient for you to come?"

If the client has stopped smoking for a certain length of time – even just a few days – but has relapsed, then say something like, "That's fine. The great thing is that you have done it – you did stop smoking for a few days" (or whatever time the client stopped for). Ask the client what the specific situation was that led them to revert to smoking, and then validate what happened. Typical events which lead to a reversion to smoking include a stressful work situation, an argument with someone, and drinking with friends who still smoke. In some cases, the client will have succumbed to physical cravings. Whatever the client's description, you pace it. If the client has gone back to smoking, you say:

> "There is no such thing as failure, only feedback. Learning to live as a non-smoker can be a bit like learning to drive a car. By practising it, we get better and better at being prepared for different situations on the road. When they first get behind the wheel of the car for their first lesson, most people don't immediately start driving like an expert. They realise that there are many things they have to learn about the realities of the road. So they continue to practise in the knowledge that they can and will master the art of driving, the more they commit to it. It's exactly the same with adapting to life as a non-smoker. What we're going to do when we meet again is repeat the success you enjoyed in the first few days, but make sure that this time, you're well prepared to stay a non-smoker in every similar situation."

If the client experienced severe physical cravings but has not actually reverted to smoking, then you say:

> "Now that you've given your body a breathing space, in which it clears out all the accumulated tar, nicotine and carbon monoxide, your body is learning to adjust to this new, healthy way of life. It takes just two weeks for the body to clear itself and become a non-smoker's body. When we meet, we will work on ways of enabling you to get control over these feelings and enable the process of adjustment to become much easier and smoother."

In some cases, the client will simply have continued smoking without a break from the moment they left your therapy room. In such cases, you say,

> "There is no such thing as failure, only feedback. It can take a certain amount of practice to learn to live as a non-smoker. Every individual has a unique pathway to becoming a non-smoker. When we meet next time, we will take a slightly different approach in order to find your way of achieving that goal."

Sometimes a client will say something like, "It didn't work," or, "The treatment was unsuccessful." In that case, you direct attention from the abstract "it" to the pronoun "I". You ask, "If you turn that around and say that same sentence beginning, 'I experienced …', how would you express it?"

The vast majority of clients are reasonable people who recognise that it is in their interests to commit to success by mastering the techniques and becoming and staying non-smokers.

Problems arise, because, hardly surprisingly, no client will have foreseen in sufficient detail all the trials they will encounter in everyday life. These can easily undo the changes.

Despite your best efforts, there may be a part of the client's mind which clings to the habit of smoking for reasons as yet unknown.

There are also those clients who resent you for taking away a cherished habit which has become part of their identity. There may even be a genuine fear of the prospect of becoming a non-smoker.

Some clients understand logically and rationally that they should quit smoking in the interests of their health, but a powerful internal impulse convinces them in advance that hypnotherapy will not work, and they retain a "distance" from the entire process during the session.

Unfortunately, the occasional client expresses hostility or blame towards the therapist for the fact that they have relapsed, or have not yet succeeded in stopping smoking. Others are highly sceptical of the whole process of hypnotherapy and its capacity to enable them to become non-smokers. Clients never blame themselves – any blame is directed against the hypnotherapist. You must remain completely committed to the client's success and retain your own certainty of their ability to become and remain a non-smoker. You must convey this certainty to your client at all times. On the rare occasions when a client becomes rude or aggressive, resist any temptation to respond in the same way. Instead, you can pace and lead them. Start by agreeing with them: "Absolutely!" This puts them in the odd position of having nothing to fight against. Then say, "So what do you want to do about it?" in order to get them to think constructively.

Dealing with the client's experience

When the client arrives for the follow-up session, continue to communicate the certainty of their imminent success in becoming a non-smoker. Say: "So, what's been happening since our last meeting?" Whatever the client says, pace their experience and give much the same message as you gave over the telephone when the client called. The central point to get across is that "Calm seas never made good sailors." You could draw an analogy with some skill which the client has previously acquired. For instance, if the client plays tennis, you could say:

> "Remember when you first started playing tennis? Probably you got a few things wrong in the early stages. Maybe you misjudged the direction and location of the ball, and knocked it over the net with the incorrect amount of force. But you assumed that you would ultimately master the sport, so you recognised that those early mistakes were part of the whole process of becoming a tennis player. It's the same with becoming a non-smoker. You can understand this reversion to the habit as a temporary mistake which you can learn from as part of the experience of quitting smoking."

Alternatively, you could substitute a learned ability which the client mentioned in the previous session, such as playing a musical instrument, learning a foreign language or mastering a complex job skill.

Then, depending on the client's experience, you can say:

> "Every time we aim to do something and it doesn't quite happen the first time the way we'd ideally like it to, we can obtain information which can enable us to find a more effective way of doing it next time. Can you remember exactly what went through your mind the moment you reached for that cigarette on Thursday evening?"

What you are searching for is the client's description of the internal subjective experience, or trigger, which led them to reach for a cigarette after having stopped for some hours or days or weeks. Having identified that, you can then make changes to it.

The DVD technique

A good way to enable clients to learn from their experience is the DVD technique. Most clients will be familiar with using DVDs.

First you want to put the client into a relaxed state of internal focus and awareness. The quickest and easiest way to do that in this context is to draw on the instant self-hypnosis you taught the client in the previous session. With almost all clients who attend for a follow-up session for smoking cessation, this memory of self-hypnosis is the most reliable means of achieving a satisfactory trance state.

So you say: "Can you remember that instant self-hypnosis we did last time?" The client is likely to say something like, "Vaguely" or, "Kind of". Very few clients actually practise it in the way you taught them. You continue, "Shall we do that now?" The client will assent by saying, "Okay", "Sure" or similar.

So you say:

"Excellent. I'd like you to once again find that point where your head feels weightless and leave it there, please. Great. Now your head is exactly aligned over your body, which means that your breathing is at its best. With your eyes closed, just be aware of your breathing. And just as you did before(breathe slowly, deeply and evenly, building up a nice, natural rhythm of deep, easy breathing. Breathing from the diaphragm, just below your lungs, where your abdomen is. That's right. And every time you breathe out, can you expel all the air from your lungs, breathing in completely new air, so that you're getting a really good air circulation? That's right. And every time you breathe out, say the word "calm" to yourself, silently and mentally. And every time you breathe out, see the word "calm" written right in front of you, written in your mind's eye. And every time you do this, you'll be putting yourself into a peaceful, calm, comfortable state.

"And in this relaxed state, your unconscious mind has full access to all of your memories – just as if you had a DVD player on which you could play DVDs showing every moment of your life. You already know all about DVD players. How you can *s-l-o-w the picture d-o-w-n* so that you can see everything in *v-e-r-y s-l-o-w m-o-t-i-o-n* [mark these words out by speaking slowly]. How you can *speedimupsoeverythinghappensveryquickly* [mark these words out by speaking quickly]. How you can freeze-frame and go backwards. How you can *zoom in really close* to capture details. And you know how on a DVD you can often listen to a running commentary from an actor or the director? In the same way, you can hear that continuous train of thought going through [name's] mind during every moment of his/her life."

Assuming that the client did in fact stop smoking for a few days, then went back to smoking during some social event, you continue:

"So put on that DVD which shows [name] walking out of this therapy room last week. And take a look at how he/she allowed the body that breathing space, expelling tar and nicotine and carbon monoxide, so that that body got healthier and fresher and more energised, hour by hour and day by day. And notice [name] waking up in the morning as a non-smoker, feeling high energy flowing through mind and body, breathing fresh, clean air into strong, clean and healthy lungs. Observe [name]'s daily routine, living as a non-smoker, at home, out and about, working, socialising, relaxing [whatever the client's daily routine actually is]. See and hear everything. And really notice the difference. And remember that you can slow down, go backwards, freeze-frame and speed up, just as you like, to really see and hear how [name] lived as a non-smoker for those days [and weeks]. And I'd like you to find the very best moment during that time of living as a non-smoker. And when you've found that moment, I'd like you to step inside [name]'s body – so that you can actually feel the way your body feels, see what you can see with your own eyes, hear what you can hear – and actually live this life you're leading as a non-smoker, and really notice the difference. And if there's any word or phrase that comes into your mind that can describe that experience, then you can say that word or phrase out loud now if you like."

What you are doing here is reframing the client's experience as a success – at least for the time when they did stop smoking. Since the client has proved that they can – and have – stopped smoking for some days or weeks, then they can repeat that success – and this time ensure that they stay a non-smoker. Also, you are tapping into an actual positive resource – the memory of living as a non-smoker. You are building up the client's optimism and confidence that they can and will indeed live as a non-smoker; the purpose of the follow-up session is simply to learn effective methods of staying that way.

The client may give you a word or phrase, such as "energised". If they do not give you a word, then offer your own, such as "healthy". Either way, you anchor that experience. Having focused on a positive experience from the days of living as a non-smoker immediately after the first session, you then move on to the specific situation in which the client reverted to smoking. If the client accepted an offer of a cigarette while drinking with friends in a pub after work on a Thursday night, then you would say:

"And I'd like you now to fast-forward that DVD to last Thursday evening, to the moment when [name] was walking down the street with those friends towards that pub – and then watch as they enter that pub and find somewhere where they can drink. Hear [name] talking, joking and laughing with those friends. Notice the flow of thoughts running through [name]'s head. And then notice how they all enjoy a drink or two and the conversation just flows. Be aware of how those friends are lighting up and offering cigarettes round. And s-l-o-w t-h-a-t D-V-D d-o-w-n now, so that you can see and hear every detail of what happens as they offer that cigarette to [name]. Notice the expression on his/her face, how he/she holds his/her body, listen to that continuous running commentary flowing through his/her head. And now, as you slow down e-v-e-n m-o-r-e, just step inside [name's] body and experience in v-e-r-y s-l-o-w m-o-t-i-o-n that moment when that friend offered that cigarette. Can you identify exactly what you are feeling, what you can see, what you can hear, what that running commentary in your head is saying – in that moment in which you accept that offer? (Pause.) And perhaps you can say now out loud what you are aware of in that moment?"

Give the client all the time they require to describe that experience. Let's say the client replies, "As Mike offers me the cigarette, I'm breathing more quickly,

I feel a tightness in my throat, and I can hear a little voice in my head saying, 'Go on, just have the one cigarette with this round of drinks.'"

Then you would reply,

"Okay. Just focus on your breathing now. And I'd like you to slow down your breathing – breathe slowly from the diaphragm, expelling all the air from your lungs, and breathing in completely new air. And turn down the volume of that little voice in your head so it's very quiet indeed. (Pause.) And can you get that voice to say instead, 'It's great to socialise and stay a healthy, happy non-smoker. It's great to socialise and stay a healthy, happy non-smoker.' (Pause.) And can you turn the volume up so that it's loud and clear? (Pause.) And can you put it in stereo so that it's on both the left and right hand sides of your head? (Pause.) And is there a piece of music that you find inspiring, that you can play as a background to that voice? (Pause.) And that feeling in your throat – can you loosen it, as if ripples of relaxation are flowing down through your throat, melting away that tension so those muscles become comfortable and relaxed?"

Give the client a few moments to make these changes. Then you can ask: "And what are you aware of now?" The client might reply, "I feel more peaceful." You say:

"Excellent. As you continue to see and hear and feel that experience, I'm just going to touch your right wrist. [Touch the opposite wrist to the one that you anchored before.] Peaceful. Peaceful. Peaceful. Peaceful. Peaceful. And any time in future that you're out drinking or socialising, or in any other situation where that temptation might re-appear, all you need to do is touch that wrist in this way and say that word to yourself again and again and you'll be well protected, so that you stay a non-smoker throughout that situation."

By using these simple techniques which draw from the client's own internal subjective experience, the client can ensure that they always have a more useful way of responding to future similar situations, and therefore of remaining a non-smoker. Note the precision with which this exercise deals. The purpose is to "zoom in" on the precise moment when the client reverted to smoking, and make precise changes to their internal representations. The greater the precision the client can attain with identifying these representations and changing them, in order to be well protected against the risk of succumbing to the temptation to smoke a cigarette, the better.

The DVD metaphor is ideal because you can indeed slow down, freeze-frame, speed up, go backwards, zoom in and, as with many DVDs, play it with a commentary by the director, the actors and so on – similar to the running commentary going on in the client's own head.

If your client did stop smoking for some days or weeks and then reverted in a particular situation as a result of a specific internal subjective feeling (stress, cravings, temptation while socialising or whatever), then say:

> "If you think about it, for twenty-three hours and fifty-nine minutes of the day you are perfectly fine, a healthy, happy non-smoker. Then for just that one minute of the day there is a temporary feeling of stress/cravings/temptation/ etc, which passes through your mind. Now if you can just let that temporary feeling pass through your mind, until a few moments later your mind focuses on something else, you will stay a non-smoker. Very often we experience a moment of stress/cravings/temptation/etc, and very soon we realise that it's all a fuss about nothing. We've forgotten about it the very next day. But those people who respond to that temporary feeling by reaching for a cigarette are simply bringing back a habit that will still be there long after that situation in that moment has been forgotten. So for that one minute out of the twenty-four-hour cycle, if you can just realise that that moment is a temporary happening and just let it pass, then very soon you'll forget that moment and you'll stay a non-smoker."

This is a reframe of the client's experience which is both more accurate and more useful than labelling the relapse to smoking as a "failure" or something which "just happened". Rather, the client is learning from what happened in order to gain greater control over their momentary subjective experiences, become a non-smoker again, and this time stay one permanently.

Moments of insight like the above, in which the client realises that it is only that one minute out the twenty-four-hour cycle that they need be concerned with, are far more decisive in turning a client into a non-smoker than the whole rigmarole of deep trance phenomena and its ideomotor responses. Very often, straight talk to your client while they are in full waking awareness will bring about those moments of insights which are key in enabling them to live as a non-smoker.

You might occasionally encounter a client who is not familiar with watching DVDs. In that case, use the photo album metaphor in which you ask the client to go back and look at a photo of the moment in which they reverted to smoking, and then make changes in the same way. Otherwise, use watching television or going to the cinema as a metaphor.

The purpose of the follow-up session is to get the client back on track, and enable them to learn more useful ways of dealing with the situation which resulted in the reversion to smoking.

If the client did not stop smoking at all after the first session, and simply smoked within an hour or so of leaving your premises, with no change to previous habits, then you simply say,

"Everybody has a unique pathway to living life as a non-smoker. Last time we met, we achieved a result different from the one we were seeking. Your unconscious mind has clung to that habit for its own reasons, which are perfectly good ones as far as it is concerned. Today, we're going to take a different approach to enabling the unconscious part of your mind to find a new and more useful way to achieve that positive intention than through the smoking habit. Remember the story about Robert the Bruce hiding in the cave? How he watched that spider attempt to spin that web again and again until the spider finally got it right? If at first you don't succeed, try, try again. But instead of the word "try", let's use the phrase "approach from a different angle". I'm sure that's what the spider did to construct that web successfully. We're doing much the same thing today."

Either way, give reassurance to the client that they will become a non-smoker – and be able to stay one – as a result of the follow-up session.

An approach for trance induction on the follow-up session

Once this preliminary exercise is over, induce trance and convey the following message. Tailor it to the specific experience of the client sitting before you. Omit any section which is not congruent with the client's actual experience, and feel free to add any elements which you think might be of benefit to them.

Draw again on the client's previous experience of self-hypnosis, as in the first session, as this repeated experience of trance will be deeper than it was before. Then say:

> "And just be aware now of all those memories, stored away in your unconscious mind, in the form of mental images, showing every moment of your life. Just like photos in a pile of old albums."

Most clients find it easy to access their memories through the photo album metaphor. The actual experience of looking through a photo album is usually a pleasant one, and something they have already done and can relate to. (By contrast, the metaphor of a filing cabinet as a repository of memories is often associated with paperwork, accounts, bills and other unpleasant chores.) However, you can tailor the metaphor to the client. With an artist, you could talk about an art gallery containing many rooms with drawings, paintings and sculptures depicting different experiences in their life. Later in the session, you could ask the client to imagine creating an artistic work which represents the transformation to becoming a non-smoker.

With a computer hobbyist, you could describe a box filled with storage devices containing all the client's memories, including tape reels, floppy discs, zip drives, CD-Roms and memory sticks. This could lead to a metaphor about the unconscious mind behaving like the malfunctioning computer HAL 5000 in the film *2001: A Space Odyssey*, and needing to be reprogrammed with new software.

> "And I'd like you to choose now that photo album which shows the last time we met – when [client's name] came to visit [therapist's name]. And I'd like you to have a good look at the photos of [client's name] in that situation – as he/she heard [therapist's name]'s voice and made sense of those words in his/ her own way. Notice as [client's name] becomes more and more relaxed with each moment. How his/her face becomes incredibly still because the muscles of the face were so relaxed. How his/her breathing becomes slower … deeper … more even. How all the muscles of his/her body become even deeper relaxed. How he/she begins to lose track of time and space. How everything *s-l-o-w-s* … *d-o-w-n* … in a pleasant … healthy … comfortable way. How his/her mind starts to wander freely, his conscious mind, that is – perhaps through the imagination or pleasant memories. While his/her unconscious mind, that creative inner intelligence, is open … active … listening … learning … ready to make a wonderful transformation."

As you describe the externally visible aspects of trance in this way, it is likely that you will see the client manifest them as they look at the imaginary photograph of the memory. Whatever the client's attention is focused on will be reflected in their physical experience. Assuming that the client did stop smoking for at least a couple of days or more, you continue:

> "And can you remember how your unconscious mind heard my words and made sense of those words in its own way. So that somewhere deep inside, that creative part of your imagination started to learn differently. That creative imagination reflected on the fact that you were born a non-smoker – that you lived as a healthy non-smoker throughout your childhood years and the early teenage years, [and into your early adult life – if appropriate]. And that creative imagination – throughout the course of your life – has already experienced a whole series of learning moments of transformation in which you learned to walk, to run, to read, to write, to drive, and to achieve so many other things that you have done in your life. [Here, of course, you can add some achievement specific to the client, such as mastering a musical instrument, achieving success in some sport, or becoming fluent in a foreign language.] Moments of transformation in which it left behind stuff that was no longer of any value to you and embraced instead new learnings which were more useful and appropriate to your life today.

> "And when we met just last week [or whenever], your unconscious mind carried out another wonderful moment of transformation, a breakthrough, an epiphany, in which it all came together. And in that moment, your unconscious mind realised that you were a non-smoker. That you could live as a non-smoker. That

that smoking habit was a temporary decision taken by the teenage/young adult [client's name] as a temporary solution to a temporary situation. That in so many ways, you've moved forward, taken on new responsibilities, left so many childish and teenage things back in the past. And in the same way, in that moment of transformation, your unconscious mind learned how to live as a non-smoker. I'd like you to look at that photo of [client's name] in that moment – notice the expression on his/her face, the breathing, the position of the head and body – step inside [client's name]'s body and repeat that wonderful moment – that epiphany – that breakthrough – now. So that once again you can let that transforming process take place within you. So that you are a non-smoker. Because that is your choice, your preference, your decision. You have no desire to smoke. Just take one silent minute to achieve that transformation now."

Remain silent for one minute. Then continue:

- "And now that you have repeated this moment of transformation, just be aware that you can ensure that you remain a non-smoker in all future situations. So that next time you go out drinking with those friends, you will stay a non-smoker throughout that experience. You can prepare yourself for the next drinking session by putting yourself into a relaxed, calm, resourceful state through instant self-hypnosis. ([If you taught the client stress management in conjunction with self-hypnosis:] And can you remember that numerical scale of alertness and relaxation, from 100 down to zero? You can change gears, going down to 20 on that numerical scale, just to give yourself the appropriate level for socialising and drinking.) You can trigger that anchor – press that wrist where I pressed and say that word "energised/healthy/etc". And if anyone offers you a cigarette, just be aware that there is a single moment of temptation, and in that moment you can weigh up all the benefits that you are now enjoying as a non-smoker: better health, much longer life, higher energy, the social advantages, the money you save, the excellent example you're setting to those you influence, how happy those people closest to you are, the greater freedom. You'll weigh up those benefits against maybe five minutes of dubious pleasure from accepting that cigarette, and you'll say, 'No thanks, I don't smoke.' And you'll let the conversation move on, and find you can enjoy those friends' company just as much as a non-smoker. And it really is as simple as that.

- "And I'd like you now to take down that photo album of [client's name]'s future life: I'd like you to flick through that album and look at the future situations in [client's name]'s life: getting up in the morning, commuting, working, socialising and drinking with friends, travelling [obviously, this depends on the client's actual daily routine], and really notice the difference. And any time you want, you can just step inside one of those photos, step inside your own body and actually live this life. See it, hear it and feel it – and really notice the difference. And I'd like to ask your unconscious mind, that creative part of your imagination, to find the best, the most powerful way to make this future a reality in your life.

Just take one silent minute to do that, starting now. (One silent minute.) And then, now that this wonderful process of transformation has become a reality in your life, you can become awake and alert and refreshed and allow your eyes to open."

Give the client whatever time they need to arouse from trance. Then you ask: "How are you feeling now?" If the client says something like, "Great", or "Energised", or "Calm", then you say, "Remember, you can feel just as good as this any time you like, if you can just find those twenty minutes a day to practise self-hypnosis."

If the client did not stop smoking at all after the first session

Some clients who return for a follow-up session did not become non-smokers during the first session. In that case, having given them the reassurance described above, you can again induce trance by repeating the "instant self-hypnosis" taught in the first session. Then continue:

"And be aware that throughout the course of your life, your unconscious mind has been guiding you forward, learning, growing, helping you to understand the world differently. When you were very small child, tucked up in bed after dark, your imagination filled the darkness around you with goblins and dragons and ghosts and monsters, so maybe you were afraid of the dark. Later on you realised that there were no such creatures out there, just the wardrobe, curtains, chairs and toys. So you could sleep soundly, leaving those imaginary creatures back in the past.

"And in so many ways, as you've grown and learned about the world and yourself, gaining more and more abilities and knowledge and experience, so your habits of thought and feeling and action have developed and adapted to become ever more useful and appropriate to the person you have become. You have been constantly adopting new habits and leaving old unwanted habits back in the past where they belong. There have been many times in your life when you've embarked on a new activity, and maybe, at the beginning, doubts passed through your mind about your ability to master it. But when you really committed to success, to learning step by step and making it happen, so it all came together. So you surprised yourself time and again by just how resourceful you are, by your capacity to commit, to learn, to make measurable improvements to every aspect of your life.

"So can I ask you to do me a small favour? Are you willing to imagine what it would be like if you did believe – indeed know with certainty – that you have the power to become a non-smoker? That just as you've successfully learned to do so many other things in your life – and just as you've left so many other things back in the past when they're no longer useful to you – so in the same way now you are learning to become a non-smoker. If you had that air of positive expectation for success, how would you hold your body? How would you breathe? How would your head be positioned? What thoughts would be flowing through your mind? What would be your expression? And will you do that for me, right here and right now? [Pause while you observe the client adopt the required physiology.] Good.

"Because you already know what it's like to be a non-smoker. You were born a non-smoker, you lived as a non-smoker as a child, as a young teenager (even as a young adult [if appropriate]). Throughout all those years, you lived healthily and happily and never once even thought about cigarettes or smoking. Your body, your brain cells, your muscles, all the organs of your body – they have memories of life during those years which are a part of your life, a part of your experience. ([If the client did previously stop smoking for over two weeks:] And can you remember how good it was when you did stop smoking, for three whole weeks/four whole months/two whole years, etc – how you gave your body that breathing space so that it recovered its proper and rightful state of health and well-being? [if appropriate].) And today, your unconscious mind is finding the way to become a non-smoker again, so that once again your body is recovering that proper and rightful state of health and well-being that you are entitled to. And now that you know all about self-hypnosis, how to put yourself into this peaceful, relaxed state any time you want, you will remain a non-smoker for ever and ever.

"So that you stop smoking – now. Stop smoking for good. Stop smoking for life. Become a non-smoker and stay a non-smoker now and forever. Give your body that breathing space it wants and needs to clear out that tar and nicotine and carbon monoxide. So that you are now a non-smoker – because it is your choice, your decision, your commitment to live as a non-smoker. And in this very relaxed state, in which your unconscious mind is listening, active and learning, I'd like to ask that creative part of you to make that choice, that decision, that commitment into a reality in your life.

"So that you will have no desire to smoke. And as you give your body this breathing space, at last allowing it to adapt to life as a non-smoker, so you know that you can handle any physical tweaks that you may become aware of during that cleansing and healing process. Those tweaks only last for ten seconds, and if you happen to experience any such temporary, fleeting tweak or pang or craving like that, then you will say to yourself:

'I recognise this feeling as a sign that my body is becoming a healthy, happy non-smoker's body. The feeling may be slightly uncomfortable for a moment, but I *can* handle it. This feeling only lasts ten seconds, and for those ten seconds I distract my attention by eating an apple, drinking a glass of water, reading the paper, or listening to the radio until that feeling passes. I know that these temporary moments of discomfort as the body cleanses itself of that accumulated poison have never killed anybody in the history of the world. I understand them as a sign that my body is getting cleaner, healthier and stronger. I *will* survive it – and I give myself better health, longer life, tens of thousands of pounds in money, more energy, social advantages, and a sense of freedom and independence by doing so.'

"And I'd like to ask your unconscious mind to take just one silent minute to reflect on everything I've said, everything you've experienced, and to find the best, the most powerful way to make this transformation a reality in both body and mind, so that once again being a non-smoker is part of your identity, just as it was during those years of childhood and early teenage life, and will be again in the future. Just take one silent minute to do that, starting now. (One silent minute.)

"And this wonderful process of learning, understanding and transformation can continue tonight, tomorrow and in the days ahead. So that as you become more and more used to life as a non-smoker, so your mind will become more and more clear and calm, while your body becomes more and more supple and relaxed. Finding your energy level rising, so that all that trapped physical and mental energy comes back at your disposal. So that you find it easier to live life resourcefully – drawing on the power you already possess within yourself to deal more effectively with the world, with the people you deal with, with every situation. Cultivating the habit of self-hypnosis, creating calmness within, finding the most appropriate level of alertness and relaxation for every situation. Finding yourself enjoying life more, taking life in your stride, opening yourself up to those things that your unconscious really wants for you deep down. And as you leave that old unwanted habit back in the past where it belongs, so you find yourself positively embracing this better and healthier future.

"And in your own time, you can become awake and alert and refreshed, and allow your eyes to open."

Give the client time to awake to full waking consciousness. Then, as before, you ask, "How are you feeling now?" This both directs the client's attention to their present state (and away from what they have just experienced in trance) and gives the client the opportunity to describe that present state. Assuming that the client gives a positive word or phrase, such as "I feel pretty relaxed", then you say,

"Excellent. You can enable yourself to become just this relaxed any time you like, through the regular practice of self-hypnosis. And it will be far better, healthier and more useful than anything artificial. So you'll be prepared for every situation to stay a non-smoker for life."

Three key ideas

If the client has either continuously smoked since the first session, or else stopped smoking for a while and then reverted, then a useful technique to use in the second session is that of asking the client to reflect on three key ideas. This is an adaptation of a technique by the father-and-son team Herbert and David Spiegel. I have adapted their original version, which is somewhat authoritarian, to something more permissive. This technique gently reminds the client that smoking is a serious problem for the body. However, it avoids making specific reference to the illnesses and fatality which smoking can cause. The strength of the technique lies in that it states three facts which the client recognises to be true, and then encourages the unconscious mind to come up with its own conclusions derived from those facts. While the client is in trance, you say:

"Everybody who becomes a non-smoker does so in their own individual way. I'd like to ask your unconscious mind to find your individual path to that healthy, happy non-smoking future. And in order to do that, I'd like to ask your unconscious mind to reflect on three key ideas which it can make sense of in its own way.

"The first idea is this: for your body, smoking is a poison – at least potentially it is damaging to that body. Now you are more than your body, but your body is a very important part of you, and for your body, specifically, smoking is a poison. (Pause.)

"And the second idea is this: you need your body in order to live. The healthier your body, the better your life. Indeed, in order to have any life at all, you need a functioning body. Your life depends on the well-being of your body – and the healthier and stronger and fitter and more energised your body, the better your life will be. Your body is a valuable and delicate physical mechanism through which you experience life. (Pause.)

"And the third idea is this: your body cannot think for itself. You have to do the thinking for it. Now you know that smoking is potentially damaging to the body, but your body doesn't know that. Your body is a trusting innocent creature that depends on your judgement for its survival and its well-being. And the wonderful thing is that you already possess within you that sense of responsibility and compassion towards a trusting, innocent creature which you can draw upon now in order to protect it. I don't know if you have a pet, maybe a dog or a cat or a bird. Or maybe you used to have a pet. Or at least you can imagine what it would be like having a pet. Now just imagine going to the pet shop and coming back with a box of pet food, and just before you were about to serve that food to your pet, you noticed a massive sticker on the side of that box which said, 'This pet food kills pets.' 'This pet food causes fatal diseases in pets.' 'This pet food seriously damages the health of pets.' Now, I ask you, would you give that food to your pet? Of course not – you'd throw it away. In fact, you'd make sure the pet couldn't get at it even after it had been thrown away.

"And just imagine if you were escorting a small child across busy streets in [name of client's town], where they drive like maniacs. You would be unusually cautious about crossing those roads when you were with that kid. You'd stand on the kerb with that child's hand in yours. You'd wait until the little green man/[Walk sign in the US] was lit, and even then you'd look from left to right to make sure the cars stopped where they're supposed to stop before briskly cross-ing that road with that kid's hand in yours. You see how your natural sense of compassion and responsibility comes into play every time you are looking after a trusting, innocent creature? I'd like to ask your unconscious mind now to just take one silent minute to find the way to apply that sense of compassion and responsibility to that other trusting, innocent creature, your body."

Pause for one silent minute to allow the client's unconscious mind the oppor-tunity to find its own path forward.

Note that this particular technique in part adopts a negative or aversion approach, with the references to smoking being a potentially damaging poison. This technique should be used with caution. It is a means to an end. It is only used in the context of a follow-up session, after the entirely positive approach of the first session did not achieve the desired result. It does draw on the client's knowledge of the deluge of anti-smoking propaganda which delivers a nega-tive message by describing illness and death. However, it seeks to "contain" and utilise that knowledge by surrounding it with positive messages about the client's resourcefulness in taking successful action to overcome the risk of such consequences. The tone of voice in which you say these references is important. Make them a subtle but clear reminder without great emphasis. To get the right tone, imagine that you are Jeeves tactfully informing Bertie Wooster of some unwelcome news. (In P. G. Woodhouse's comic stories, Wooster is an upper-class twit who is constantly being helped out of difficult situations by his clever butler Jeeves.)

A story about stopping smoking

Another technique suitable for use in the follow-up session, if the client has either stayed a smoker or reverted to the habit, is that of telling a story about a previous client of yours who successfully stopped smoking. People relate to stories, and in particular to characters similar to themselves in those stories. The goal here is to describe a previous client of yours who is similar in gender, age and lifestyle to the present client, and tell the story about how they success-fully quit smoking. The client you describe can be a real client, a composite of two or more actual clients, an invented client, or a mixture of fact and fiction. We will use an example here of a male client who is a police officer, married and with children. Let us assume that he enjoys playing sports, and has attained accomplishment in them, and that he started smoking as a police cadet. Once you have induced in the client a state of internal focus through repeating the "instant self-hypnosis" taught in the first session, you could say:

"So that as you enjoy this pleasant relaxed experience, you can just be aware of all the things that you've learned at an unconscious level – and all the things that you've left back in the past which no longer have any relevance to you.

"And I'd like to tell you a story about a gentleman who worked in the fire service who came to see me because he wanted to become a non-smoker. He had been smoking for a long time. When he first joined the fire service, the training was pretty demanding. In a new town, with a new bunch of friends, taking up smoking became a way of being part of the group when they all went out for a drink after a tough day's training. But after he qualified as a firefighter, as the years went on, he felt that smoking habit becoming more and more of a burden on his body. Because he had to keep in shape for dealing with emergencies, he knew that his body's performance wasn't quite what it should have been. He decided to quit smoking when he got married, and he did quit, for a while. But somehow he drifted back to smoking. And when his wife told him she was expecting a baby, and she quit smoking, he quit too, but again somehow he found himself going back to that old habit again. Maybe it was stress, or going out drinking with a bunch of smokers, or boredom, or some unexpected problem which led him to go back. Whatever it was, by the time he came to visit me, he was fed up of smoking. He wasn't even enjoying the cigarettes any more. And as his children grew taller, so he felt more and more that by quitting smoking permanently he would be setting so much of a better example to them. So by the time he came here, he was more or less ready to break free of that habit – and to stay a non-smoker for good.

"He sat right there opposite me, and as he heard my words, he entered a very relaxed state. His breathing became deep ... and slow ... and even. He became aware of the most relaxed part of his body, and let that feeling of relaxation flow through the part of the body next to that, and the part beyond that, until all the muscles of his whole body were completely relaxed. He found that his conscious mind was wandering, and he sort of lost track of time, just like one of those pleasant Sundays at home when he didn't need to do anything at all. But his unconscious mind was listening and learning and making sense of everything I said and he experienced.

"Because that unconscious mind had been helping him to learn, helping him to grow, every since he was a very small boy. When he first learned to swim, he had those little artificial floats on his arms. But the more he practised swimming, the more he could stay afloat without the artificial floats. And then his unconscious mind enabled him to learn the doggy-paddle … the breast stroke … the front crawl … the back crawl … the butterfly … until pretty soon, he could simply dive into that pool and swim length after length without even consciously thinking about it.

"And when he joined the fire service, that same unconscious mind helped him to learn so many skills. He reached a peak of physical fitness, learned to work as part of a team, learned to stay calm and resourceful in the middle of a fire. He could enter a burning building and rescue someone trapped inside and take it all in his stride. That's because his unconscious mind made him a fireman.

"And when he came to see me, that same unconscious mind was listening, learning, absorbing my words and making sense of them in a way which had meaning for him. The unconscious mind which had been protecting him and guiding him forward, ever since the day he was born, turned him into a non-smoker in a single instant. He experienced a breakthrough, an epiphany, a moment of transformation, in which it all came together. In that moment, he imagined that he could see and feel every cell in his body. And those cells began to expel all the poison that had been trapped inside them. His body expelled tar from the lungs, carbon monoxide from the bloodstream, and nicotine from every part of his body. He imagined he could see clouds of thick, smelly, filthy, disgusting black smoke being expelled from his body as that bad stuff flowed out of it, and he knew that his body was getting fresher, cleaner and healthier by the moment. Then he saw stinking, foul, corrosive, awful grey smoke being expelled, and he knew that more and more of that poison from way back when was leaving his body for good. At last he saw white, transparent steam being expelled, and he knew that all of that horrible poison had left his body for good and his body had achieved its rightful and proper state of health, freshness and well-being. (Pause.)

"And it really was as simple as that. His unconscious mind freed up all that physical and mental energy that had been trapped by that old habit. He went out of here feeling optimistic and energised. He lived daily life, working, travelling, socialising, enjoying home life and family life. He found his energy level increased, his senses of smell and taste recovered, and his enjoyment of life improved in every area. His focus of attention shifted to the worthwhile, beneficial, desirable things in life. He welcomed the fact that he had greatly extended his life, greatly improved his long-term health prospects. He felt at ease with himself and with the world. He knew how happy his family was that he had made this transformation, and what an excellent example he was setting to his children, knowing that they were far more likely to grow up to be non-smokers, now that he was himself a non-smoker. He simply forgot about that old habit. That habit was simply left back in the past, where he had left eating jelly, and kids' cartoons, and those swimming floats and so many other things which no longer had meaning or value for him. And he has stayed a non-smoker ever since.

"And I'd like to ask your unconscious mind to take just three silent minutes to reflect on all this. Three silent minutes to make sense of it all in your own way. Three silent minutes to carry out this same wonderful transformation. Three minutes to make it happen, starting now.

(Three silent minutes.) "And this process of learning, understanding and transformation can continue today, tonight, tomorrow and in the days ahead. And in your own time, you can become awake and alert and refreshed, and allow your eyes to open."

In this technique, the key is to describe a previous client who has some similarities to the actual client sitting in front of you, without being too close a match. If the previous client you describe is too similar, the present client is likely to realise that and become self-conscious that you are talking about them. So talk about someone with similarities, but also with enough differences to be recognisably a distinct person.

In this example, where your client is a policeman, you are describing your previous work with a firefighter – an occupation with many similarities in terms of training, camaraderie and ability to deal with emergencies. The client's unconscious will connect powerfully with these similarities. Because your client enjoys participating in sports, he will relate to the description of learning how to swim, even if his preferred sport might be rugby. You could conceivably even be tapping into an element of friendly rivalry between the emergency services, as when the police and fire service play each other at football or cricket. The client might unconsciously think, "Well, if a bloke from the fire service can do it, I'm sure not going to let the police side down." Your description of the firefighter's family life will also have obvious resonance with the present client. Thus your client will be fascinated and absorbed by the story, and manifest its message in his own life.

If the client in front of you is, say, a grandmother who has recently retired from a career in bookkeeping, and enjoys growing flowers as a hobby, then you might talk about a lady client whom you recently helped stop smoking at the time of her retirement as a secretary, and how she had much more time for growing vegetables once she became a non-smoker. You could also mention the excellent example that a previous client is setting to her grandchildren by becoming a non-smoker.

By telling a story about some client who is similar, but not identical, you are tapping into a fundamental trait of the human psyche. Your client has come to you to become a non-smoker. They may have doubts – at least at a conscious level – about whether they can do it. As you tell your story about how some-one similar to them did it, your client cannot help but connect to that character in that story. The doubts in the conscious mind are bypassed, and the uncon-scious mind is free to realise the ideas in the story and turn the client into a non-smoker.

When the client is still a non-smoker during the follow-up session

Some clients will have successfully stopped smoking but request a follow-up session because they want to be able to cope more easily with the process of adjustment to life as a non-smoker.

Welcome the client. Occasionally, they might express the view that they are imposing on you by coming back for a follow-up. Respond by saying, "Not at all. We're here to make sure that your transition to the non-smoking life is as smooth as possible, so it's a great pleasure to be able to work with you again."

Then ask, "So what's been happening since our last meeting?" The client then describes how they have stopped smoking, but have experienced difficulties – which may be physical cravings or emotional or psychological issues – in adjusting. For example, the client might say,

> "On Wednesday I faced an incredibly stressful day at the office, and in the mid-afternoon I felt like a cigarette and went outside to get one, but then made myself turn round and go back inside. I haven't actually smoked yet, but I feel that I could go back to it any day now, so I thought I ought to come back and see you."

With such a description, it is essential to validate the client. You say something like,

> "Many congratulations on your success. You've proved that you can do it, and you have done it. What we're going to do today is make sure that you've got more useful ways of dealing with these stressful situations, so that you can create calmness whenever you want it."

Then you can use the DVD technique described above to get the client to go back and re-examine in detail that stressful moment in the office on Wednesday. As mentioned previously, you teach the client self-hypnosis again in order to provide a more useful way of dealing with future situations of stress, and apply it specifically to a future-paced situation at the office. Then you give some ego-strengthening suggestions and awaken the client.

There may be a high degree of repetition, both of specific techniques and of the overall "message" in this follow-up session. This is absolutely fine. It is more effective to re-use techniques and ideas which the client has already responded to successfully than to introduce them to new and unfamiliar techniques. The client is more likely to be comfortable with material which is familiar to them.

The "emergency stop" technique

It is always a good idea to use the "emergency stop" technique in the second session. Say, "What we want to do now is what's called the emergency stop. Would you say that you're an experienced driver?" If the client does not drive a car, then adapt the wording to cycling or even walking.

> "And whenever you go on the roads, you want to know that you've got excellent brakes, so that you can apply the emergency stop any time you really need to. You hope you don't face a situation where you need to do that, but if you do, you're well prepared and know exactly what to do.

> "And whenever you're on the road and you see a red traffic light in the distance, you find your foot pressing down on the brake without even needing to consciously think about it. And it's the same when you see one of those big round metal 'stop' signs they put up in front of roadworks – you slow down without needing to think about it. What we're going to do now is to draw on that experience in order to make sure that you always have a way of protecting yourself instantly in case you ever get caught off guard in the future.

> "I'd like you to imagine that you're sitting in a cinema, in front of massive wide screen. And can you do that more easily with your eyes open or *closed*?"

At this point the client is likely to close their eyes, but if they stay open, that is fine. It means that the client can do this particular exercise more easily with the eyes open. Sometimes a client will ask specifically, "Do you want me to close my eyes?" If so, reply: "Closing your eyes simply cuts out the visual field, so that you can focus your attention entirely on what's going on inside. So if it helps you see that wide screen more easily, then you might like to let those eyes close."

Whether the client's eyes close or remain open, continue:

> "That's right. And on that screen, there's a red traffic light, big, bright and clear, and filling the whole screen. And can you superimpose over that picture, in a double exposure, one of those great big red stop signs they put in the middle of the road – a red disc with the word 'STOP' in white letters – so you can see both the red traffic light and the 'STOP' sign at the same time? (Slight pause.) And

I'd like you to superimpose over *that*, as a triple exposure, a policeman, glaring right at you with a stern expression on his face, his arm outstretched, his palm upwards. And hear that policeman saying in a very stern, authoritative tone of voice, the word 'stop … stop … stop … stop'. Hear that loud and clear in Dolby stereo as you watch that triple image of the red traffic light, the red 'STOP' sign and the policeman. And at the same time, hear the squeal of the brakes and feel the juddering of the car as it comes to a halt. And now I'm going to touch your right wrist."

Now you are going to place an anchor on the client's wrist. Make sure that you use the other wrist than the one you used in the first session. Touch the client's right wrist and say the word "stop" several times in a stern, authoritative tone of voice. "Stop … stop … stop … stop … stop." Then remove your hand from the client's wrist. Continue:

"And now, as you go out in the real world and live this new life, so you know that just as you have the emergency stop in reserve every time you're driving, so too you will always know how to apply this same emergency stop any time you may need it in the future." (If the client's eyes are closed:) "And in your own time, you can become awake and alert and allow your eyes to open."

After demonstrating the "emergency stop", you ask the open-ended question, "Anything else on your mind that you want to mention?" as at the end of the previous session.

At this point you end the second session, congratulating the client on their success and again emphasising the importance of focusing on the positive.

Chapter 10

A checklist for one-to-one smoking cessation

Success in hypnotherapy, especially for smoking cessation, depends on getting every detail right. With smoking, there is no scope for "partial success" or "slight improvement", as might be the case with weight loss, pain control, confidence or countless other issues. Every smoker who wants to quit the habit has two conflicting impulses. Part of the client wants to stop smoking, understands the benefits of doing so and is motivated to make it happen. The client has powerful unconscious resources which seek to protect their health – resources which you will draw upon in the session. However, another part is clinging to the smoking habit and will seek any rationalisation to keep smoking, however absurd it might seem. The client can justify clinging to the smoking habit, by using any "mistake" or any "reason" as a pretext: the hypnotherapist's shoes were scuffed or dirty, the bathroom was a mess, the pens didn't work or there was no box of tissues. They extrapolate from what they see to negate the entire process of hypnotherapy. Once a client has rationalised an apparently trivial thing which went wrong, or of which they disapproved, they may lose confidence in the entire process and remain a smoker.

Once such a thought enters the client's conscious mind, it is difficult to make the session a success. Therefore, by going through the following checklist before and after each session you will be doing everything in your power to eliminate the possibility of such thoughts and leaving nothing to chance.

Needless to say, there is no need to limit yourself to what is on this checklist. Some hypnotherapists buy fresh flowers for their consulting room every day. By all means add such touches if you feel they are feasible and desirable.

Checklist

		Yes	No
Before the session			
1	When the client booked, did you sent a personalised letter on headed paper, signed in blue ink, preferably by first-class post (or else by e-mail) giving the location, time, day and date of the appointment?		
2	Have you included a short written description of what the client can expect during the session (teaching self-hypnosis, accessing resources for unconscious transformation, learning to live as a non-smoker in daily life, receiving a CD and handout)?		
3	Have you included a map with directions of how to reach you, with information about parking and public transport?		
4	Is the exterior of the building as user-friendly to the client as can reasonably be expected? (For instance, has any clutter been removed? If the client is due to arrive after sunset, are the entrance and the buzzer or doorbell properly lit?)		
5	Is the room in which the therapy is to take place clean and tidy? (Also, is the hallway through which the client passes en route to the therapy room clean and tidy?)		
6	Is the temperature in the room comfortable? (In cold weather, has the room already been heated before the session? In hot weather, is there already a fan, air cooler or air-con unit switched on, functioning and reasonably quiet?)		
7	Is the form to be filled in by the client already printed out and on the table or desk? Are there at least two functioning pens next to it?		
8	Are the CD(s) and the handout to be given to the client at the end of the session already on the table or desk? Do you have business cards easily available?		
9	Is there a box of paper tissues within reach of the seat where the client will sit?		
10	Are bottled water and two clean glasses present in the room for both the client and yourself if required? (Optional: are tea, coffee and fruit juice available if you choose to offer them? If so, make sure that you have fresh milk, sugar and artificial sweetener, and that you can make and deliver the drink quickly.)		
11	Are you ready to accept payment from the client and issue a receipt if requested? Do you have change for a cash payment?		
12	Have all telephones, alarms, pagers and other noise-making devices in the therapy room been switched off? (The exception is the phone number you have given the client. Keep this phone switched on in case the client is running late or lost. When the client arrives, switch it off.)		

		Yes	No
Before the session (continued)			
13	Has everyone in the building been informed that the session cannot be interrupted under any circumstances whatsoever?		
14	Is everything in the bathroom spotlessly clean, tidy and at a comfortable temperature with a dry floor? (Has it been pre-heated in winter?)		
15	Is the lavatory functioning and flushing correctly?		
16	Is there a more than adequate supply of toilet paper?		
17	Is the water from the hot water tap in the basin actually hot enough for washing hands and face?		
18	Is there soap on the ledge of the basin (preferably from a liquid dispenser rather than a bar)?		
19	Is there a clean, dry towel on the towel rail?		
20	Is the client's route from the therapy room to the bathroom clean, tidy and easy to follow?		
21	Have you made yourself generally neat in appearance? (For instance, has your hair been combed?)		
22	Is your clothing spotlessly clean and neat? (For instance, are the shoes shined, shirt ironed and pet's fur removed from jacket? Do both socks match?)		
23	Is your watch functioning and accurate (and any alarm, radio or musical function switched off)?		
24	Are you and the entire premises completely ready for the session at least 15 (and preferably 20 or 30) minutes before the appointed time?		
25	Have you practised self-hypnosis before the client's arrival?		
26	If the appointed time comes and the client has not yet arrived, has the therapist (working from home) gone outside the front door and looked for the client?		
When the client arrives			
The remaining items need to be checked off at the end of the session.			
27	Have you greeted the client warmly?		
28	Have you built rapport by engaging in small talk with the client while en route to the therapy room?		
29	Have you offered to take the client's coat and any bags? (If so, have you put them away quickly?)		
30	Have you sat the client down behind the desk and had them fill out the form?		

		Yes	No
During the session			
(This section does not have to be adhered to exactly, because each client is different and some questions may not be relevant to all clients. Sometimes you may be pressed for time and unable to complete all the points.)			
31	Have you asked the client how they started smoking?		
32	Have you explained that every problem was once a solution, and that the purpose of the session is to find a new and more useful way of achieving that positive intention?		
33	Have you explained the "nicotine trick"?		
34	Have you asked the client whether they have stopped smoking for any length of time in the past?		
35	Have you asked the client about their recent smoking?		
36	Have you sought to use submodalities to change the client's subjective temptation to smoke?		
37	Have you explained to the clients about ultradian rhythms?		
38	Have you asked about smoking to change mood (e.g. stress)?		
39	Have you taught the client instant self-hypnosis, incorporating stress management if the client requires it?		
40	Have you asked the client about their experience with the self-hypnosis exercise and responded to their reply?		
41	Have you prepared the client for the main situations to be faced in which the temptation to smoke might recur?		
42	Have you told the client about how to deal with a "moment of temptation"?		
43	Have you prepared the client to deal with the issue of cravings?		
44	Have you prepared the client to deal with the question of the transfer of energy?		
45	Have you dealt with any issues specific to the client, such as weight and eating, socialising and drinking, or marijuana?		
46	Have you induced trance in a way which connects with the client's experience (past or present)?		
47	Have you got all the essential messages relevant to the client across in trance?		
48	On awakening, have you asked the client about their present state and dealt with it satisfactorily?		
49	Have you given the client the "benediction" of advice at the end of the session?		
50	Have you given the client the handout and CD with instructions on how to use them?		
51	Have you congratulated the client and invited them to return for a follow-up session if they so desire? Have you given the client your business card?		
52	Was payment taken smoothly and quickly?		

		Yes	No
The follow-up session			
Obviously, your premises have to be just as well prepared for the follow-up as for the initial session. The following questions are specific to the follow-up session.			
53	In the preliminary phone conversation, have you reframed the client's experience and given reassurance of success for the follow-up?		
54	Once the session begins, have you asked the client for a description of their experience and dealt with it?		
55	Have you used techniques relevant to the client's experience, e.g. the DVD technique?		
56	At the end of the session, have you checked your work to ensure that the client has achieved the result sought? If the client reverted to smoking in some situation before the follow-up session, do they know exactly how to stay a non-smoker in that same situation?		

Chapter 11

Various tips for one-to-one smoking cessation

Assume success

Assume that the client is already a non-smoker, and that it is merely a technical matter of mobilising the client's unconscious resources and educating them in the techniques to stay a non-smoker. Clients respond to your sense of certainty at both a conscious and unconscious level. Conversely, even the slightest doubt on your part will be picked up by the client either consciously or unconsciously, and will undermine the client's prospects, perhaps fatally – both figuratively and literally. Expectations tend to be realised.

Visualisation, affirmation, projection

The late Ormond McGill exhibited remarkable speed, intensity and effectiveness when he used hypnosis on subjects. He explained that he used a technique called "visualisation, affirmation, projection" to powerfully affect his own state, which the subject picked up on – perhaps unconsciously – and responded to.

First, hold an image in your own mind of what you want the subject to do. See a picture of the client doing what you want. Second, make an internal affirmation telling the client to do whatever you are visualising. Third, imagine "projecting" or "throwing" that picture towards the subject and say that affirmation out loud in the form of your suggestion.

Communicate in positive terms

Most official anti-smoking propaganda focuses on the negative. We see horrific descriptions of smoking-related illnesses, print advertisements showing the horrible muck which accumulates in a smoker's body, and commercials showing funerals of smokers who died before their time. Even that old 16mm film was negatively biased. Also, people who are encouraging their relatives, friends, patients and so on, to stop smoking often communicate in similar terms, however well-meaning their intent.

The problem is that people often screen out negative messages and experiences. They also resent the bearer of bad news, associating that person with the news they are bringing. When smokers are blamed for being weak-willed, or accused of being stupid or irresponsible, their instinct is to become defensive and challenge the person making these claims. The smoker's unconscious mind then blocks out the message. Negative anti-smoking messages, therefore, tend to induce an unresourceful state in the smoker. Experiencing a state of fear or self-disgust, or both, is precisely the opposite of the positive resourceful state in which one's ability to become and stay a non-smoker is mobilised. Many clients for smoking cessation will indeed arrive in a negative frame of mind. When you get a client who experiences fear, self-disgust or defeatism, your task is to get them to a more positive, optimistic state of resourcefulness. Orientate the client's attention towards the positive resources and achievements which can be associated with their past and future healthy life.

Communicate in positive terms, as far as possible, and educate the client to think in equally positive terms. Talk about the better health, longer life, greater energy, more money and better skin that the client will enjoy as a result of becoming a non-smoker. Even the phrase "becoming a non-smoker" is a relatively positive communication and is preferable to "stopping smoking" or "quitting smoking". It implies a new identity to replace the client's previous self-identification as a smoker. Although the word "non-smoker" still includes "smoker", it has no synonyms which omit that word. The most useful way to get around that slight drawback is to listen to the client's descriptions of what their life will be like – or was like – as a non-smoker. They might use words or phrases such as "healthy", "more energised" or "pleased with myself". Make a mental note of these and feed them back to the client as the client's positive representation of what the smoke-free life means to them.

However, when they fill in the form, many clients express themselves in negative terms when they list the benefits they are achieving by becoming non-smokers. When you feed back those values to the client during the trance, reframe them in positive terms. If a client writes, "I don't like the fear of getting lung cancer," then rephrase that as, "You think about how great it is to enjoy that confidence in your body's ability to maintain its health, now that you are a non-smoker." If the client writes, "Hate the horrible smell in home, clothes and fingers," then you can rephrase that as "You appreciate how your sense of smell has returned to its proper level, so that you enjoy the fresh, clean smell in your home, on your clothing and on your fingers." If the client writes, "No longer a social outcast," then you rephrase that in positive terms as "You think about how good it is to enjoy the social advantages, so that you can go anywhere, socialise with anyone and enjoy this wonderful experience of social acceptance."

If the client says, for instance, "I keep beating myself up because I'm so weak that just I can't stop smoking," reassure and validate them by saying something like,

> "Many people get into thinking that way. But the reality is that when you started smoking, you did so for a good reason. The unconscious part of your mind accepted the smoking habit as the best way to achieve the positive intention it was seeking for you when you were a teenager. Until now, it's continued with that habit. Today we're asking the unconscious to develop a new, more useful way of achieving that positive intention, and once it does that you will become a non-smoker. When people beat themselves up and label themselves as weak, and assume that they can't stop, they're creating a pattern of thinking, feeling and acting that is likely to keep them smoking. So what we are going to do now is a simple exercise in self-hypnosis which will give you a more useful way of thinking about yourself – as a strong, creative, resourceful individual who is accessing the power to learn to live as a healthy, happy human being."

This is a form of ego-strengthening. With smoking cessation, it is not merely useful, but more or less essential to boost the client's ego and convince the client that they have the capacity to live as a non-smoker.

In practice, it is not possible to communicate in positive terms all the time. Direct suggestions such as "stop smoking" and "you have no desire to smoke" are in a sense negative, but they are justified because you have to make totally clear to the client what you want them to do.

In this respect, smoking cessation differs from the other issues with which the hypnotherapist deals. In a therapeutic session when I am seeking to help a person experiencing depression, for example, I never use the word "depression" or its derivatives. Instead, the client is asked to provide a word to describe the state they want to achieve, which could be "happiness", "joy", "wellbeing" or "optimism". We then focus all our efforts on mobilising the client's resources in order to achieve that desired state. The state the client wants to get away from – the D-word – is not mentioned. However, with smoking cessation, the smoking habit is "the elephant in the room" which both client and therapist both know is there and has to be dealt with.

Communicate as simply as possible

Communicate to your client in the simplest possible terms, so that they can understand and connect with everything you say. When inducing trance, use the method which is simplest for your client (not necessarily for you). Make your inductions as effective as possible by tailoring them to the experience of the individual client sitting in front of you. Use the words they use, and talk about their enthusiasms and interests. This may mean adapting your approach to connect with the client. When you ask the client to do an exercise, such as visualisation, changing submodalities or self-hypnosis, simplify the process as much as possible. Only ask the client to imagine one thing or perform one task at a time. Methods which require changing two or more visualised pictures at the same time may frustrate and lose the client.

Avoid long-drawn out techniques. A technique that is short and to the point will quickly produce benefits for the client. You are the one who has to be flexible. Remember the three-second rule. If the client is not connecting with a particular technique, give it a maximum of three seconds, then say, "That's fine", and move on to another approach.

Personal mastery

To do hypnotherapy well, you need to study, memorise, practise and repeat the techniques to the point where they are automatically available to you during the actual therapy session without having to consciously search for them. Once you have achieved that level of unconscious mastery, you can adapt the entire session to your client's life, communications, experiences and resources, connecting what you see and hear to your wealth of unconscious knowledge of hypnotherapeutic techniques. Eventually you will reach the point where you can carry out an entire session without being consciously aware of what is coming next. Although you are learning plenty from courses, books, DVDs and so on, it is the clients who really teach you mastery. It is with the "awkward sods" – the more challenging clients – where your skill as a communicator is tested to the limit and you really learn how to handle every situation.

Make the client the "star" who is carrying out the transformation

Attribute the power, skill and success to the client, rather than to yourself. The client is the expert on their life, their habits and their future. The hypnotherapist's skill is in activating and mobilising the client's "hidden" resources and educating the client in how to use them effectively. Adopt the attitude of "the customer is always right". If you find yourself getting impatient with or exasperated by a client, remember that you are still learning – and that to become a "good sailor" you need those rough seas. You are being tested: are you able to access your own resources? In accepting your own humanity, you are acting as a role model for the client.

The better you are able to call upon your deepest resources, to benefit from the hard work you have put in to learn how to be the best hypnotherapist, the more will rough seas become fun to navigate, and the easier it will be to set a course over uncharted oceans. A committed navigator can sail in any conditions in any water. A committed hypnotherapist, therefore, accepts every client who wants to attend for smoking cessation (and who is willing to pay the fee). Positively welcome those clients who describe themselves as "difficult cases", "repeated failures", "addictive personalities" or suspect that they "can't be hypnotised", as you will learn the most from these people. The clients have placed such labels on themselves, so show them how to change or reframe them with new and more useful ones.

You could invite the "difficult case" to recall an experience, perhaps passing an exam, when they thought it would be difficult but in fact it became easy. With a client who claims to be a "repeated failure", reframe that as a positive resource:

> "You've already successfully been through that experience of becoming a non-smoker and living as one. We can ask the unconscious mind to repeat that experience and this time make sure you're prepared for every situation to stay a non-smoker permanently."

Ask the "addictive personality" to substitute the word "habit-forming" instead. This is a simple reframe. Point out that everyone takes up and abandons many habits throughout their life, and that it is nothing new or special to leave behind the particular habit of smoking and adopt the habit – or "addiction" – of enjoying high energy, excellent health, good skin, social advantages, freedom and all the other benefits that come from life as a human being free from that old, abandoned habit.

Even if the client comes across as poorly motivated and cynical, the very fact that they have turned up and – presumably – paid the fee proves that there is a part of them that wants to become a non-smoker. Do your very best to strengthen that part and make it decisive, always assuming that the result you seek will be achieved.

You may be pleasantly surprised in many such cases when you learn that the client has indeed become a non-smoker. Even if they have not, you have still gained knowledge that you will not find in any textbook, or even from working with an "easy" client.

It is impossible to predict accurately who will and who will not become a non-smoker. So take everyone who comes to you, and always presuppose success.

Chapter 12

Building a one-to-one therapy practice

Sergei Rachmaninov was asked what sublime thoughts had passed through his head as he stared out into the audience during the playing of his concerto at Carnegie Hall in New York. "I was counting the house," he said.

Nearly 85 percent of people who train in hypnotherapy in the UK go out of business within twelve months because they do not get enough clients. A common mistake is to spend large sums on advertisements in the press. These are almost always a waste of money. The abundance of published material on how to do effective hypnosis with clients once they arrive is matched by a dearth of material on how to get clients in the first place. Any book for hypnotherapists about smoking cessation which did not provide some useful information on effective, low-cost methods of building a practice would be incomplete.

This chapter offers some guidelines on how to build your practice, and how to avoid the common traps into which many have fallen. Necessarily, it largely concerns itself with the financial questions that have to be faced by hypnotherapists as they offer their services to the public.

Running a commercial business

To achieve financial success as a lay hypnotherapist, remember that you are running a commercial business. We take money from members of the public in return for the services we offer them. We have to think and act like businesses in order to survive. We are subject to the same laws and regulations relating to advertising, legal liability, fair trading, access to premises, financial transactions, regulatory obligations and countless other areas as any other industry. As far as the law is concerned, the fact that we consider ourselves to be caring, ethical, humanitarian and so on, makes no difference.

No contradiction exists between maximising your income and your commitment to helping people improve their lives. Quite the reverse: the more you charge, the more value you can give your clients. The more money you accumulate, the more you can build capital to invest in longer-term projects which may require considerable financial layout, and take time to come to fruition, but can reach more people and enable them to improve their lives.

These projects include events such as seminars and smoking cessation classes, which cost significant amounts to organise and promote; products such as CDs, DVDs and printed publications; and the whole lengthy and sometimes expensive process of reaching the corporate market. All these involve spending time and sums of money with no guarantee that for any individual project you will get a return on your investment. Never spend money you cannot afford to comfortably say goodbye to. The more capital you can accumulate from helping people, the more you can finance bigger, longer-term projects which in term help larger numbers of people.

The effective hypnotherapist tends to develop a unique approach to therapy which is somewhat distinct from that of all other therapists. While they all draw on what has proven to be effective in practice, each therapist is a unique individual whose approach derives from their own experiences, beliefs, preferences and values. You might like to consider that a medium- to long-term goal of your practice is to ensure that your services are made available to as many people as possible in formats and at prices that are comfortable to them.

With smoking cessation, you could run one-to-one sessions in your own home at one price for local people, and another for individual sessions at a clinic where a higher fee could be set. You can run smoking cessation groups for the public, which people can attend for a lower cost than a one-to-one session. If you offer smoking cessation seminars for the corporate world, your services can be made available to people at their workplaces, with the cost paid partly or entirely by the employer. If you produce a product such as a smoking cessation CD or DVD set, then people anywhere in the world can order your product and benefit from your therapy at low cost.

You are running a business in which your goal is to maximise your financial income. This can only be realised by consistently helping people achieve what they desire to the best of your ability. Find ways to make your services in smoking cessation – and indeed in other areas – convenient and affordable to as many people as possible in as many formats as possible.

Project the right image

All voluntary financial transactions happen because someone chooses to pay money to a second person in the belief that the goods or services offered by that person are worth the money.

People are perceived as worthwhile if they come across as strong, capable and successful. Everything you say and do, and all your publicity material, must support the image you want to portray. That image has to reflect the reality of your ability to get results and give value for money.

In an article in *Harpers and Queen* in 2004, the artist and writer Lady Liza Campbell described how she was seeking therapists who could enable her to get control over her finances. Lady Liza wrote:

> "Then I got an email inviting me to Holistic Connections, a forum for the professionally spiritual. I met astrologers, colour counsellors and aromatherapists – and life coaches. I took away three business cards, with a view to taking each of them on a metaphorical test drive.

> "The next day, I eliminated one because, on closer inspection, his business card was decorated with pale pink rabbits and a winking elf. The second bit the dust when, during a phone call, she told me she was 'completely skint at the moment'. I wouldn't jump into the back of a taxi with a driver who had just told me they have no sense of direction; so why would I put my trust in a life coach who was advertising her own life as being as shambolic as mine?"[1]

Attempts to make silly jokes on your publicity material, or announcing yourself as being financially unsuccessful, are sure-fire ways of repelling prospective clients. Have a business card which is simple raised black or blue text on white card. If you *are* "completely skint at the moment," do not tell that to potential clients who are seeking your services in order to get control over their finances.

Charging the right fee

> "There is scarcely anything in the world that some man cannot make a little worse, and sell a little more cheaply. The person who buys on price alone is this man's lawful prey."
>
> John Ruskin

A small-scale independent trader – whatever field they are in – can hardly ever afford to compete on price with large-scale operators. With smoking cessation, one-to-one hypnotherapy is a unique individual tailored service, not a mass-produced commodity like nicotine replacement therapy (NRT) products, and the price you charge inevitably reflects that. It is a mistake for a hypnotherapist to try and attract clients by offering the lowest-cost service in the area. Such an approach usually means cutting corners in terms of quality and time devoted to your clients. It is far better to strive to achieve the best possible results for your clients, and to aim to constantly improve your service by adding as much value as possible.

Aim to be one of higher-priced hypnotherapists in your area – as well as *the* most effective and dedicated to the success of your clients. Visit the websites of hypnotherapists in your area (usually displayed in their ads in the Yellow Pages), and see how much they charge. Position yourself in the top 10 percent in price – and make sure that you are at the very top in quality. With the smoking issue, specifically, the lifetime financial savings the client will make by stopping are vastly out of proportion to the cost. Nevertheless, be realistic about what local people can afford.

Be prepared to go the extra mile to benefit your client by providing additional services beyond those you have agreed. For example, should a session go on beyond the scheduled ninety minutes, then I keep going for as long as it takes – sometimes up to two-and-a-half or even three hours. Conversely, if we finish the whole smoking cessation procedure with twenty minutes to spare, I will use that remaining time to help the client with any small issue they might have mentioned as wanting help with, such as building confidence or sleeping better. You may also give the client other material that you have produced, such as CDs, articles or booklets. Make sure your standard charges cover the costs involved in providing any little extras.

Bear in mind the psychology of pricing. *Provided that your service is indeed effective*, a relatively high price tells potential clients that the additional value they are receiving justifies the higher price. Helping people stop smoking through hypnotherapy is a demanding and complex skill. Price it too low and your clients will not take it seriously. Price it relatively high for the local area, dedicate yourself to excellence in achieving your clients' goals, and both you and your clients will benefit.

Nine hours marketing for every hour with a client

In the early stages of your practice, you will have to spend at least nine hours marketing for every one hour you spend with a paying client.

The financial rewards from one-to-one therapy are by their nature somewhat limited. When you do one-to-one therapy with individual clients, you encounter a fundamental business problem. A general maxim of business is that it takes six times as much effort and expense to acquire a new paying customer as it does to sell to your existing satisfied customers.

In businesses such as office supplies, pizza delivery, dry cleaning or accountancy services, satisfied customers return again and again for more of the same.

Therefore, most businesses which are satisfying their customers' needs do not need to make great efforts to reach new potential clients in order to survive. They can increase revenue more easily by selling more and different goods and services to their existing satisfied customers.

With one-to-one hypnotherapy, and particularly for smoking cessation, the opposite is true. The more quickly and effectively you satisfy your clients' needs, the faster you lose those clients. A client attends a session with you, becomes a non-smoker and no longer needs your services. Because you have been successful, you never see them again. True, the same person might return to deal with another issue, and might – or might not – choose to refer others who become paying clients.

However, this word-of-mouth strategy is a haphazard, unpredictable and passive way of expanding a practice. To build up a regular practice, you have to go out and make the effort – repeatedly – to get new clients. Your flow of clients will be irregular. Certain months – usually July, August, December – are generally quiet for one-to-one hypnotherapy, particularly for smoking cessation. You can get around these fundamental business problems by planning, as early as possible, where you are going to go in your career beyond doing one-to-one therapy. Now many hypnotherapists are quite happy just doing one-to-one therapy and have no desire to go further. However, if you want to maximise your income, while building up your one-to-one practice, then you should simultaneously be taking action to move towards those areas where significantly greater revenue can be generated: group sessions which individuals pay to attend, and corporate sessions which enable employees of a firm to become non-smokers *en masse*. Another potentially profitable area is turning a service into a product – creating a short-run booklet, CD, DVD or similar product which embodies your knowledge in concrete form, and which the purchaser can use to achieve their goals. Of course, these products are likely to be for other issues besides smoking. It can be a time-consuming and expensive process to set up the group sessions and get people to pay to attend them, to promote your seminars to the corporate world, and to create your products and sell them, but in the long term they will generate far more revenue than one-to-one.

As you build your practice, not only will you be focusing on getting and dealing with one-to-one clients, you will also be setting up events and creating products, and you will be promoting them more or less simultaneously.

"It's always easier to write a cheque"

A general maxim of marketing tells us that the more you pay, the less effective the method. The more the method depends on the amount of work you put into it, the more effective it will be. Advertising which you pay for (especially at the card rate) is – generally speaking – the fastest and most efficient way to waste money ever invented. By contrast, the most effective ways of attracting paying clients are those methods which take a fair amount of work on your part but which involve little or no financial outlay. Remember the saying: "It's always easier to write a cheque." Many people – not just hypnotherapists – assume that by writing a cheque for advertising they are getting value for money by delegating the task of recruiting customers to the newspaper or magazine. Nothing could be further from the truth. To achieve real success, you have to put in the promotional efforts yourself, at first hand. You cannot pay someone else to do your push-ups.

Be unique – not a commodity

Your central purpose in marketing your practice is to position yourself as being a unique solution, not a commodity. When hypnotherapists promote themselves in media such as directories, Internet listings, the Yellow Pages and paid advertising, where they appear alongside numerous other hypnotherapists, the potential client has little or no way of differentiating them. In such a context, price tends to become the determining factor.

Therefore, focus your marketing efforts in contexts where you come across as "the only game in town". It is far more effective to come across as a live person than merely a piece of paper or an Internet web page.

There are numerous groups in your area, including service clubs, business groups and public libraries, which would welcome you as a speaker at their events. Providing demonstrations of hypnotic phenomena, some of which are described in the next chapter, will impress audiences and convince them that there is "something in it". The more talks you give in your community, the more you will get known.

Send news releases to the local press and radio stations about what you are doing to help people become non-smokers. In the UK, National No-Smoking Day is on 14th March every year. Local press and broadcasting outlets cover activities in their area relating to smoking cessation, and this can be an opportunity for you to gain media exposure. You can also write articles for newspapers, magazines and websites on subjects related to what you do. Examples of such articles could be: "Smoking cessation in the workplace," "How to influence your children to avoid smoking," or "Managing stress after you quit smoking." Keep clippings of all press articles written by or about you, and put them up on your website. Such media coverage tends to increase your credibility.

Money-back guarantees

Should you offer a money-back guarantee to clients who attend smoking cessation sessions?

Before giving the arguments for and against the idea of such a guarantee, let me explain that when I started out practising hypnotherapy in my own home, I did not offer such a guarantee. When I first trained in Ericksonian hypnotherapy, my two main interests were rapid psychotherapy – helping people improve their lives in just a few sessions – and mind-body healing. In the first years in practice, however, far more clients attended for the classic issues of weight loss, confidence, freedom from phobias and above all smoking, than for these special interests. When promoting my hypnotherapy to conventional medical facilities, such as doctors' and dentists' surgeries, hospitals and pharmacies, and giving talks to groups, the question of smoking cessation came up far more often than any other issue. So I ended up devoting far more time to the smoking issue than to any other.

When I set up in Harley Street in 2000, I had to get clients through the door very quickly in order to cover the high costs. Because the overhead there is expensive, I had to charge clients a correspondingly high fee. To justify this high fee, I used the concept of "risk reversal": the supplier of the service, not the customer, takes all the financial risk. Usually, in smoking cessation with hypnotherapy, the client takes the financial risk. The client wants to stop smoking and is seeking services which enable them to do that. Not knowing much about hypnotherapy, the client is supposed to accept the hypnotherapist's claim that they can cure the client of smoking, and the client pays money to the hypnotherapist for that service. As there are numerous hypnotherapists to choose from in any given town, this means that unless the client has been specifically recommended to a particular hypnotherapist, the only criterion for selection becomes price. But if you compete on price, you die on price. It is a sad fact that most of the hypnotherapists who set up on Harley Street do not get enough clients to make it cost-effective, and have to abandon their practices there after a few months, having lost money in the process.

So I make an offer which puts no financial risk on the client. On my leaflets and website, and in a classified ad in a weekly listings magazine, I offer the client a 100 percent money-back guarantee of success. If, after the hypnosis session, the client reverts to smoking within three months, their fee is refunded in full.

In order to claim a refund, the client has to call me before the three months are up. Then, at the end of the three months, the client takes a test on a Micro CO machine, which measures the amount of carbon monoxide in their breath, and determines from that whether they are a non-smoker, a light smoker or a heavy smoker. If the machine proves that the person has reverted to smoking, their fee is refunded in full.

To make payment as easy as possible, I offer clients the opportunity to pay in instalments on any schedule they desire. For instance, the client could pay four instalments a week apart, or three instalments a month apart, or whatever fits their cash-flow best. The offer emphasises that the client can arrange it so that they would be paying less per week or month for the hypnotherapy on instalment than they were previously spending on cigarettes.

This offer of a money-back guarantee undoubtedly increases the number of clients. You are making the client an offer with no down-side: either the client gets all the benefits of stopping smoking, or should they revert to smoking, they get the entire fee refunded. However, offering a money-back guarantee is not recommended for all hypnotherapists in all circumstances. It is suitable for those in specific situations such as when I was setting up in Harley Street and had to build a practice from scratch with paying customers quickly. It is not recommended if you already have an existing hypnotherapy practice with a reasonable number of clients coming in.

There are several drawbacks to offering a money-back guarantee:

(1) A significant proportion of clients will indeed revert to smoking within three months. Some will claim a refund without wanting to come back for a follow-up session. Others will attend for a follow-up and still go back to smoking and claim a refund. So it can cost you money. To make it viable, you have to increase your fees to those clients who successfully become non-smokers. In other words, those who commit to and achieve success pay more to subsidise the unmotivated who refuse to master the techniques and apply them in the real world.

(2) A money-back guarantee creates a perverse incentive to the client to revert to smoking. People respond to incentives and are repelled by disincentives. If there is a money-back guarantee, the client has a strong financial incentive to revert to smoking within the guarantee period. In a situation which offers the temptation to smoke, the thought is likely enter the client's mind: "If I smoke a cigarette now, I will get an immediate financial reward of £x in cash. So what if I go back to smoking? This whole process of trying to stop with hypnotism has cost me nothing, and I can always go on the patches at some time in the future. Maybe next year or some time like that." So the client smokes the cigarette and claims the refund.

(3) The offer of a money-back guarantee tends to attract precisely the type of smoker who really wants to stay smoking, and who may be going through the motions to please someone else, such as a spouse, parents, employer or

doctor, who is encouraging the smoker to quit. Such a smoker is likely to sit through the session and either stay smoking or quickly revert and claim a refund. They can then say, "Well, I went to see a hypnotist to quit smoking, and I'm still puffing away. Looks like I'll always be a smoker." Taking this attitude has cost nothing, as the fee has been refunded.

(4) With those clients who are partially motivated, the money-back guarantee will tend to work against their resolve to stay a non-smoker. Even if they came to you convinced at a conscious level that they wanted to quit, in the case of any difficulties in adapting to life as a non-smoker, the awareness of that chance to get their cash just for smoking one cigarette will always be present – and an incentive to revert to the habit.

(5) The existence of the money-back guarantee sends a message that the hypno-therapy might not work, thus creating a degree of doubt in the client's mind about the prospect of successfully becoming a non-smoker.

(6) The hypnotherapist has no control over what the client does once they leave the premises. However capable you are, however well you carry out your role in preparing the client for the non-smoking life, the client has the power to undo your work on a whim, or for no reason at all, with no financial cost to them. Indeed, the client will receive a cash reward from the therapist for doing so. Unfortunately, there are a few callous people out there who actually relish the exercise of that sort of power.

(7) It is possible that in a particular month a large proportion of clients – perhaps even a majority – will revert to smoking, thus leaving you with a substantial financial liability.

So unless your circumstances call for it, I would not recommend giving a money-back guarantee. If I were to suddenly withdraw the money-back guarantee, that might produce more problems than it would solve. So before you make any offers at all, you need to think through the consequences very carefully.

However, it is still essential to offer the client back-up in the form of a follow-up session, if they require it. Some hypnotherapists offer what they call a "lifetime guarantee", in which the client can return for as many sessions as they like, but money is not refunded. That is certainly a realistic option, but even then, be aware that some clients might take that as an signal to spread out the therapy – which could be done in just one or two sessions – over five or ten. When facing a situation where the temptation exists to have "just the one" cigarette (that is, to return to the smoking habit), the client is likely to think, "Well, if I take this cigarette, I can always go back to that hypnotherapist at no extra charge to be freed from the habit again. May as well have some fun by smoking in the meantime." Absurd, of course, but that is smoker's logic for you. Needless to say, in theory, at least, this could happen every weekend for the rest of your client's life.

Therefore the best option for most hypnotherapists is to make a formal offer of the main session, plus self-hypnosis CD and written handout, plus one follow-up session, with no money-back guarantee. However, if, after the follow-up session, the client calls you and requests a third session, you can either informally give that third session for free (despite it not being a part of the original offer) or else charge a small sum for it (much less than your regular therapy fee).

Your decision about money-back guarantees depends on your individual situation, experience and preference. However, once you have chosen your approach, ensure that it is clearly written up in your leaflets, on your website and in your letter to the client, so that the client understands the terms and conditions.

Chapter 13

Running a group smoking cessation event

From individual to group smoking cessation

Once you have had at least two years' experience with successfully helping clients to stop smoking in one-to-one hypnotherapy, you will be in a strong position to organise group smoking cessation events which people pay out of their own pockets to attend. The advantage for attendees is that they can become non-smokers at your group events for a much smaller fee than for one-to-one therapy. The advantage from your point of view is that once you build up the numbers attending, you can receive a great deal more money from a group event than from working with individuals.

Be aware that running groups takes much time and effort, and considerable expense. You have to ensure that everyone in your locality who would like to stop smoking knows about your group events, and you have to convince them that those events will indeed enable them to become non-smokers. Get in contact with local newspapers, radio and television stations, and websites providing local news, and send them press releases about your group event. Ask permission to put up notices or leave leaflets in buildings where local people congregate. You could even arrange for a leaflet delivery company to deliver flyers about your events to every address in a particular area.

The first key point is to commit to success in the medium and long term rather than to expect instant riches. The second is to start on a small scale and gradually build up. Your strategy with regard to smoking cessation groups should start with finding a small and affordable venue where you can work with a few people, repeating the event at regular intervals (say, one evening every month). As word spreads about the good results you are getting, over a period of months and years, you can expect larger numbers to attend.

It is likely that the early group seminars will either lose money or just break even. However, in the long term, as you repeat these seminars year after year, you may become something of a local institution and will be able to generate steady revenue from these groups. You would be in good company. The late Allen Carr made millions from running smoking cessation groups, starting in his own home, and his formula is now being taught in clinics around the world.

Creating the right atmosphere

Once you have your venue, it is best to ensure that it looks packed. You do not know in advance exactly how many people will register, let alone how many will actually show up. If you can find a local building with several rooms of different sizes, such as a college, hospital, hotel or town hall, then ask the venue manager if you can make a flexible arrangement in which you can book the room most appropriate to the numbers who actually attend. This would be a room which looks full, but which can fit everyone in with a few seats to spare for any late or unexpected arrivals.

If possible, get people to pre-register (and preferably pay in advance) so that you have a good idea how many are going to be there. You can be reasonably sure that nearly all of those who have already paid will be there. Among those who have not paid in advance, at least a quarter who booked will not show up. However, some people may arrive without having booked, so be able to take payment from them on arrival. In order to encourage pre-payment, you could have one price for pre-payment (for instance, £20) and another for payment on the door (for instance, £30).

When people arrive, have a table where your assistant takes each attendee's name and hands over a brochure and self-hypnosis CD. Apart from the CD's obvious purpose in enabling the person to listen to it when doing self-hypnosis in future, it also gives a sense of value for money. Also, the brochure can contain promotional material for your corporate smoking cessation service, other events you may be organising and any products you offer. You can also sell products and have reports and leaflets available on the table for anyone who wants them. In case of any latecomers, your assistant can swiftly direct them to an empty chair while encouraging them to be silent.

Have your assistant ask the attendees to fill in your form in which they state the three main benefits they are gaining from becoming non-smokers. The purpose, as in one-to-one therapy, is to get them focused on those positive benefits, and away from the habit they want to leave behind.

The goal is to create a memorable experience and inspire those attending. The positive advantage of running a group is that you can build up a powerful and inspiring group dynamic and sense of common purpose among the attendees. You can start doing this as soon as people arrive by putting large posters announcing the event all around the room and – if the management allows it – in the hallways as well.

Some people dislike the use of PowerPoint slides. If you have a strong distaste for them, then by all means do your group session without them. My own preference is to use them. Whatever is displayed on the screen tends to command the visual field. If the messages and images on that screen are congruent with the words being said, they tend to reinforce those words. A visual aid gets the essential message of each stage across to the attendees, and acts as an aide-memoire for the therapist. A different slide should be displayed at each stage of the event. Particularly with a large group, PowerPoint can help maintain high energy in the room. There is no need to confine yourself to the traditional bullet points and charts. A cartoon or photograph may get a particular point across powerfully.

My preference is that as soon as people enter the room, they see a slogan, such as "Welcome to the first day of your non-smoking life", displayed on the screen at the front of the room. The purpose is to influence them even before the session officially begins. Have inspiring, upbeat music, in a major key, when people arrive. My own preference is for Baroque music, but you could use dynamic modern ambient music (Vangelis or Mike Oldfield are popular choices). It is remarkable how such simple sensory devices, congruent with the purpose of the event, influence the mood of the attendees in the direction you desire.

Make sure that the environment is welcoming. Many public buildings are notoriously cold and draughty. If your event takes place in spring, autumn or winter, ensure that the heating is adequate. It may be necessary to visit the room hours before the session begins and ask management to borrow a mobile heating unit. Conversely, in hot and humid summer weather, ensure that large fans are in operation if the room has no air conditioning. Provide bottled water and plastic cups for everyone.

In a large room, use a public address (PA) system. In a small room, with a group of less than ten, a PA system is superfluous and looks a bit silly. It is best to use a system which is lightweight, compact and portable. If you are not technical when it comes to sound equipment, bring in someone who is and who can look after the technical side of it. Make sure the sound system is working correctly *before* any attendees arrive. The use of a PA system in a large room not only means that everyone can hear you clearly, but also the microphone becomes a symbol of power, and indeed an hypnotic object of fixation. The amplification of the hypnotherapist's voice focuses the audience's attention on that voice. In a large group, when you invite questions and comments, have your assistant take a wireless mike to each individual who wants to speak. Repeat or summarise the question so that everyone can hear it – this also gives you time to plan your response.

You can choose either to greet every individual personally as they arrive, or to remain "off-stage" until the moment the event begins and then suddenly appear as the "star". My preference is to greet everyone as they come in. It helps build rapport and lets people know that they are getting individual attention. Also, people who might want one-to-one help with an issue other than smoking are more likely to feel able to approach you privately afterwards.

Open formal proceedings by having your assistant welcome everybody and then announce you. Then walk on and address the group. With a small-to medium sized group (up to about twenty), make sure you establish eye contact with everyone there at some point. It is recommended to stay on your feet throughout the event, as this maintains an atmosphere of high energy.

Building up a group dynamic

The format of a smoking cessation group session is similar in most respects to that of a one-to-one session. Your goal is to ensure that every participant both becomes a non-smoker in the session and knows how to stay that way permanently thereafter. In order to do that, strike a balance between addressing the group as a whole and ensuring that each individual receives the attention they need. Play up the strengths that come from a group situation. When a group of people engage in a common activity for a common purpose, a form of "contagion" develops, leading to the manifestation of a *group mind*. The hypnotherapist's task is to utilise this group mind and ensure that its energy is directed towards gaining a successful result for every individual.

There are several ways of maximising the influence of this group mind. Before the session begins, put out the chairs in a semi-circle facing the therapist, so that each participant can see the therapist directly and can see the other participants in peripheral vision. The music which is playing when the participants arrive literally gets each participant on the same wavelength, as the brainwaves respond to the sounds in the environment. The brightly lit PowerPoint slide on the screen, with its optimistic message, is a visual focus for everyone's attention which will get them thinking somewhat alike.

Make the session interactive. Ask the attendees to describe how they started smoking, how they have stopped before, and what issues they want particular help with, such as stress management, weight control and socialising with smokers. They will find that they have a great deal in common. When you teach a technique, ask the participants how they experienced it and help anyone who found it difficult. Encourage everyone to speak at least once during the event, in order to build a sense of unanimous involvement.

One method of maximising the effectiveness of the hypnosis is to invite a participant who has been responding well to the techniques taught in the early stages of the session to come to the front. You can then do a simple demonstration of hypnotic technique on them and explain what is happening. Once the other attendees see and hear what is "supposed" to happen in hypnosis, they are far more likely to respond similarly when they experience it themselves.

Another way is to carry out a series of hypnotic suggestibility tests on the entire group. The purpose of such tests is more to get everyone actively involved and build the group dynamic than to test suggestibility.

Just before you either teach a technique or induce trance, move your eyes across the group, establishing eye contact with every attendee. Then look directly in front of you. This will lead each individual to think that you are looking directly at them.

Towards the end of the event, after the attendees awaken from trance, you can get them to raise their right palm upwards as if making the scouting salute, and then repeat after you a declaration of faith that they are prepared for every possible situation and will remain non-smokers for life. Although this can be done in a slightly tongue-in-cheek style, it is still a powerful group ritual which will have a positive unconscious impact.

Content of the group smoking cessation event

Your group sessions will reach maximum effectiveness if you write a script for them in your own words, and present it in a way which suits your personal style. The following section is intended to give you ideas from which you can select in order to create your own group seminar. A variety of techniques follow; it is not necessary to include everything. However you choose to organise your own group events, make sure that you have thoroughly mastered the material so that delivery is smooth and you can place your full attention on the participants and their needs.

Phase 1: Opening

Walk boldly towards a spot in front of the group. You could say, "Good evening, [name of town]. Let's have a show of hands. How many of you here tonight have been to one of my events before?" (Hands are raised.) "Okay. And how many people here knew who I was before tonight?" (Hands go up.) "And how many couldn't care less one way or the other? Yeah, I thought so."

You will probably get a laugh at this point. This opening gets the attendees involved immediately by being asked to raise their hands. The attempt at humour aims to induce a relaxed state in attendees and build rapport with them by defusing the idea of the hypnotist being "high and mighty" and the process of hypnotherapy one of "domination".

Using much the same approach as with an individual client, you then speak briefly about how people start smoking and how hypnotherapy enables them to stop. Ask attendees what they have written down as the benefits they want to achieve by becoming non-smokers. Almost all mention health, and at least half mention the money saved. The remaining reasons can range from a sense of independence, to improved sports performance, dislike of the smell of cigarettes, the social advantages and setting a good example to one's children. As the attendees find how much they have in common, this builds the group dynamic. If anyone has written down reasons as negatives, such as, "fear of developing cancer", "being a social pariah", or "horrible smell", then reframe them as positives: "confidence in my body's long-term health," "enjoying socialising anywhere with anyone", or "having my sense of smell come back so that I can enjoy the fresh, clean smell in my clothing, hair, fingers and home". Explain how the unconscious interprets everything in positive terms, and has difficulty in processing a negative. Make a mental note of these positive benefits, so that you can feed these benefits back to the attendees later, when they are in trance.

Praise your audience by talking about the power of their creative imagination and how they have already learned to do so many tasks by transferring from the conscious to the unconscious. Talk about how they are about to do the same in becoming non-smokers. Your goal here is to seed the idea of stopping smoking and staying that way permanently. Mention that in a matter-of-fact sort of way right from the start, and at each stage during the event. This seeding is unlikely to turn anyone into a non-smoker by itself. But it opens up the idea at both conscious and unconscious levels. As you go through the different exercises, interact with the attendees and then induce trance, continuously "seeding" the idea of the participants becoming and staying non-smokers, a chain reaction is set up which will bring about the transformation everyone is consciously seeking to achieve.

Phase 2: Explaining about unconscious learning

Ask the group whether anyone has been hypnotised before. You are likely to get at least one who has either experienced one-to-one hypnotherapy, attended a group hypnosis session or volunteered in a stage show. The very fact that that individual has chosen to attend your group hypnosis event implies that their previous encounter with hypnosis was a good one both in the event itself and with the results attained afterwards. So ask the attendee to describe what they experienced during the process and the results achieved from it. The purpose of doing this is of course to increase the expectations of the other members of the group; hearing about the benefits from hypnosis from other attendees has a powerful effect.

Whether any attendee has previous experience with hypnosis or not, talk about how we experience hypnotic trance every day:

"Every morning, just before we awaken, and every night just before we drift off to sleep, we are in an hypnotic state. It's a very creative state, and what we are going to do later on at this event is to guide you into that state and extend it for much longer, so that you can learn what you're here to learn. By a show of hands, how many people here have had the experience of driving on the motorway [freeway in the US], and it seems as if five minutes have gone by, but it's actually been two hours? Or if you're stuck in heavy traffic, how it seems the other way round? That's what we call time distortion – one aspect of hypnosis.

"Hypnosis is all about learning. You know what it's like when you learn some new task. When you first learn to ride a bicycle, you're consciously aware of everything. You're wobbling all over the place, struggling with the pedals and the brakes, maybe falling down a few times, until little by little you learn to keep your balance, and pretty soon you can ride that bicycle for hours and hours without even thinking about it consciously. That's because the unconscious part of the mind has learned how to ride that bicycle and has taken over the process of cycling. Your conscious mind is freed up to enjoy the scenery. In other words, the knowledge moved from the conscious to the unconscious mind.

"The unconscious mind includes all your memories, your beliefs, your values, your associations, and your habits. It includes everything going on inside your body which you don't need to consciously think about – your heartbeat, pulse, immune system, digestion of food, breathing and countless other functions, all coordinated, but outside of our conscious control. The unconscious has an intelligence of its own – it operates at the level of mind and meaning.

"This is exactly what happened when each person in this room took up the habit of smoking. The unconscious mind took up the habit because of the meaning of the smoking habit. Eighty-two percent of people who smoke today started as teenagers, the other 18 percent as young adults. They started because of the meaning, the associations, of the habit of smoking. Smoking meant being part of the gang, being grown-up, proving oneself to other young people, rebelling against authority, being cool, glamorous and sophisticated. It was those associations which attracted people to the habit, not the cigarette itself. Later on in life, the smoking habit changes its meaning: it can become a crutch, a friend, a moment to oneself, some "me time". The habit remains the same, but the meaning changes.

"The cigarette itself is just a bit of nasty, poisonous tobacco with paper round it, on fire at one end. Anyone who has taken up the habit of smoking since the mid-1960s knew when they did so that smoking is a killer. They have been told about the diseases and early death it causes in schools, in advertising, by their doctors and other health professionals, by their employers and in the media. Yet still tens of thousands of young people take up the smoking habit every year. It's the positive associations that cause them to take up smoking and stick with the habit for year after year after year.

"What we're going to do today is change that meaning and those associations. Your unconscious mind will learn a more useful way of obtaining those same positive benefits. The meaning of that smoking habit will also change: to something which you took up a long time ago in a particular situation when you were a lot younger and had so much more to learn about what's really important in life. So that you can simply forget about that old habit. Your unconscious mind is finding a new and healthier way to attain those same positive benefits. And you will learn a series of techniques to stay a non-smoker for life."

Phase 3: Hypnotic demonstrations

The next task is to build credibility in the process of hypnotherapy. Even though the participants have chosen to attend the event, some may still be sceptical about the reality of hypnosis. Practical demonstrations have the dual purpose of proving to the attendees that hypnotherapy is valid and of building the group dynamic by getting everyone actively involved. Such involvement helps to break the state the attendees were in when they entered the room, and leads them towards a more creative, inner-focused and participatory state. Involve your audience by giving them practical demonstrations of the power of suggestion. This can be done with the following three effects:

a. **Hand-circle experiment.** Say: "Now I'd like you all to do this. Raise your right hand, like this. (Raise your right hand above shoulder height and near your face, as if taking the scouting oath.) Now spread out your fingers, like this. (Spread your fingers.) And make a little gun. (Extend your right index and middle fingers, folding the others.) And make a circle. (Touching right thumb and index finger together to form a circle.) Look at the circle. Look back at my face. Place the circle on your chin. (At exactly the time you say those words, place the circle on your right upper *cheek* just below your eye. Most people will copy your movements.) You see, your chin is down here. (Point to your chin.) That's the power of suggestion.

b. **Arms rising and falling test.** Move right on to the next test without a pause. Say: "Now, will everybody please stand up?" (Once they are all on their feet, continue:) "I'd like you to extend your arms out in front of you, like this." Extend both your arms out in front of you, fingers outstretched, palms facing downwards. "Good. Now close your eyes, and keep those eyes closed. Excellent. Now keep your left palm facing downwards, and turn your right hand palm upwards. That's right. Now as you stand with your arms outstretched and eyes closed, imagine that in your right hand you are holding the handle of an empty metal bucket. One of those old-fashioned red buckets with the word 'fire' on the side. And just imagine that dry sand is being shovelled into that bucket, one shovel at a time, so that that bucket gets heavier and heavier with every moment, pulling down and down on that right hand. (Verbally mark by speaking deeply and slowly, in a "heavy" tone.) And be aware now of your left hand. And just imagine that your left hand is tied to a helium balloon by a long piece of string. See the colour of that helium balloon now. And as that helium balloon rises upwards, just feel it pulling your left hand upwards, upwards, upwards. (Verbally mark this by adopting a higher pitch and "lighter" tone.) While into that bucket on your right hand, wet sand is now being shovelled in on top of the dry sand, so that that bucket's getting heavier and heavier and heavier. And your left arm is so light that it rises up, up, up into the air." (You can repeat these suggestions until most of the audience has their arms noticeably apart. Then:) "Now keep your hands exactly where they are right now. And open your eyes. Look around the room and notice how different people have responded differently to the power of suggestion." You will find that the large majority of the audience have achieved a noticeable degree of separation between the hands. Actually, you have helped the process along a bit by getting the audience to turn their right palm pointing face upwards. This of itself causes the right arm to lower by about one inch, due to the physics of the human body.

c. **Magnetic fingers.** Continue: "Okay, now remain standing and relax your arms. And now clasp your hands together, like this." (Clasp your hands together in front of your mouth.) "Now raise your forefingers so that their tips are about an inch apart from each other, like this." (Raise your index fingers so that their tips are about an inch apart.) "Now just imagine that there are two powerful electro-magnets on the tips of both of those fingers. And imagine that the magnetic force of those magnets is pulling those fingers together tighter, tighter, tighter … Turning up the electrical power on those magnets now so they come together closer and closer and closer. That's right." You demonstrate with your own fingers so that everyone gets the message. Within a few seconds, virtually everyone's forefingers will be touching. This effect actually is more a manifestation of the physics of the human body than of suggestion. However, what you say is, "Excellent. Every single person here has now learned how to successfully respond to the power of suggestion. The electro-magnets are switched off now. You can release your hands now and let them relax. And everyone please be seated."

d. **Eye catalepsy and hand glued to head.** An optional extra demonstration is to select one member of the group who has responded particularly well to the above demonstrations. A female attendee is preferred, but not essential, for this particular demonstration. Ask your volunteer to sit in front of the group. Once she is seated, you perform a simple induction which is essentially the "instant self-hypnosis" you will later ask the entire group to carry out. Ask the volunteer: "[Name], are you ready to be hypnotised?" Once the volunteer either nods, or says yes, continue: "Good. Just be aware of your breathing now. And let your *eyes close* any time they want to."

If the volunteer's eyes close at this point, just say, "That's right." If they do not close, then place your hand about one inch in front of her eyes and say: "Just look at this hand, and follow downwards with your eyes, letting them close tightly." Then move your hand downwards below her eyes. Almost certainly, given that the volunteer has responded well to the previous demonstrations, her eyes will close as they follow your hand downwards. This is the natural movement of the eyes in such a situation. In the unlikely event that the eyes remain open even after this, then just say, "Close your eyes."

(If they remain open even after that, you have picked the wrong subject as a volunteer. But all is still not lost. Simply suggest the opposite of what you want her to do: "Open those eyes wider – wider and wider – more and more open. Look into that light in the ceiling. Make sure that those eyes stay open and do not blink and do not close them, no matter what. Keep those eyes wide open. Don't blink them, don't close them, no matter how tired your eyes get. Do not close those eyes!" Repeat along these lines for as long as necessary. Here you are creating a "double bind". If she obeys your suggestion and keeps the eyes open, then they will tire and want to blink and close, especially as she is looking at a light. If she disobeys your suggestion, she will close her eyes in order to do so, which is exactly what you want her to do. However, it is most unlikely that you will encounter such a difficult volunteer in these circumstances.)

Once the client's eyes are closed, continue: "And keeping your eyes closed, breathe slowly, deeply and evenly, building up a nice natural rhythm, filling those lungs from the bottom to the top. That's right. And with every breath you take, keeping your eyelids closed, roll your eyeballs upward to look at your forehead every time you breathe in, and relax them downward to the front every time you breathe out." Look at the client's eyeballs under the lids to check that she is doing as requested. If she is, then continue: "That's right." Then you turn to the group and say, "When she rolls her eyeballs up to the top of her head, she is creating alpha waves in the brain, entering a creative learning state." Then turn back to the volunteer. Continue:

"And every time you breathe out, can you expel all the air from your lungs, breathing in completely new air, so that you're getting a really good air circulation? That's right. And every time you breathe out, say the word 'calm' to yourself, silently and mentally. And every time you breathe out, see the word 'calm' written right in front of you. And every time you do this, you'll be putting yourself into a peaceful, calm, comfortable state. And as you continue to breathe in and out, seeing and saying the word 'calm' with every breath, and as your eyes continue to roll upwards and downwards with every breath, so you're entering that creative state where you can bring about a wonderful transformation.

"And in a moment, I'm going to touch a point on your forehead which the yogis of India call the Third Eye. And when you feel my finger touch your Third Eye, when you next roll your eyeballs upwards, I want you to look at that point and keep your eyeballs up there, looking at it. Nod your head if you understand."

Once the client nods, say: "Good." Then watch the eyes, and when the eyeballs roll upward, gently touch the centre of the volunteer's forehead. Check that those eyeballs stay looking upwards. Continue:

"Good. Keep watching the Third Eye. And you try and open your eyes, but you can't. Your eyes are shut tight. Try – try hard but you can't open them. Your eyes are tight shut."

Provided that your subject is cooperative, she will try to open her eyes but will not be able to. This "eye catalepsy" is an hypnotic phenomenon of response to suggestion. However, the effect is helped along a little bit by the physics of the human body. When a person's eyelids are closed and the eyeballs are looking upwards, it is physically impossible to open the eyes. Provided that your client does not lower her eyeballs to look forward and then open her eyes, you will get what looks like an impressive result to the other members of the group. As soon as you have demonstrated this "eye catalepsy", remove your finger from the forehead and continue:

"Excellent. Now relax your eyeballs, lower them, and let that flood of relaxation flow down through every muscle in your body. And in a moment, I'm going to pick up your left hand and put it on the top of your head."

Pick up the subject's left hand and place it palm downwards, flat on her head. The left elbow will be sticking out at an angle. Now adopt an assertive tone of voice as you move your hand up her arm from the shoulder to the hand:

"And now your arm is getting rigid, rigid and hard like an iron bar. And that hand is being welded, glued, fixed, merged into the top of your head as you feel me press down on it."

Firmly press the hand down onto the top of the head as if "welding" it onto the head.

"That arm and hand are as rigid as a statue's. That hand and that head are now one."

Check that she is indeed pressing down with the hand. Then turn to the largest and strongest-looking male in the group and ask: "Sir, would you mind stepping up here, please?" Once the man is standing next to the subject, point to her forearm and say, "I'd like you to try and pull that forearm. Try and remove that arm from her head." The man will grasp the forearm and pull, but will be unable to remove the arm. Ask him, "Can you try it with both hands? Try, try hard." Again, even with both hands, he will be unable to remove the arm. After a couple of seconds, say to the man, "That's fine, stop pulling. Thank you for your help, and please return to your seat." As the man returns, point to the subject with her hand still on her head, and tell the group:

"Ladies and gentlemen, that's the power – the energy – the strength – that lies inside every one of you. That's the power that we're going to tap into which will enable you to stop smoking and stay stopped for good."

Then you go over to the subject and loosen the hand and arm by gently moving the wrist left and right, while saying, "Just loosening there. Relaxing and loosening. Just like a rag doll. That's right." Gently place the subject's arm down by her side and then speak to her. "In a moment, you'll hear me count from one to three and snap my fingers. When you hear me say the number three and snap my fingers, you will awaken, open your eyes and feel alert and refreshed. One, two, three." Snap you fingers. "Thank you. Please return to your seat. Let's show our appreciation to our volunteer here." The group should give a round of applause.

In fact, the demonstration of the pressure of the hand on the head is again more to do with the physics of the human body than hypnosis. If a person's hand is pressing downwards on their head, then it is physically impossible for even the strongest man to lift it by holding the forearm. The purpose here is the effect it has on the attendees. It convinces them that there is "something in it" – that hypnosis works and that they all have remarkable powers to transform their lives. It is a metaphor, or representation, of the powerful inner transformation which occurs through unconscious learning. It fulfils the same function as the conjuring tricks used by shamans and witch-doctors in traditional societies. As a vital part of the healing, they appear to pull out a toad, spider or beetle from the patient's mouth and throw it to the ground. This creature represents the disease being removed from the patient. Of course, it was previously hidden in the healer's hand. This "magic trick" becomes part of the meaning of the healing ritual and experience in the eyes of the patient and onlookers. Exactly the same purpose is fulfilled with this demonstration.

Phase 4: Asking about experiences of life as a non-smoker

The next phase of the session follows the structure of a one-to-one session. You ask the attendees how they started smoking, and explain how every problem was once a solution. Talk about the "nicotine trick" – how smoking a cigarette merely relieves the effect on the body of the nicotine from the previous cigarette, and how by simply allowing the nicotine to leave the body, the trick is beaten. Almost certainly, different attendees will have experiences in common. Your role here is to chair the discussion by encouraging participants to speak, while being aware of time constraints. There may be one individual who likes the sound of their own voice, and who may need to be gently and politely encouraged to keep their comments brief and to allow others the chance to speak.

You ask for a show of hands as to how many in the group have already stopped smoking for at least two weeks at some time in the past. Probably about half will have done so. Explain how that experience is a powerful resource, and that the unconscious mind has memories of that experience which can be recovered through hypnosis. For those who have not stopped smoking since the day they started, explain that they, too, have memories of years of living as non-smokers as children, as teenagers and in some cases as young adults, and that that experience, too, can be recovered through hypnosis.

Here you are educating the attendees and building up their expectations, as well as implicitly reframing the smoking experience as an aberration in the overall context of their lives. As they realise that they did live perfectly happily as non-smokers for a good length of time, they increasingly accept the idea of achieving the same result again.

Phase 5: Making changes to the subjective experience of smoking

Ask the attendees how many cigarettes they have been smoking per day recently, and in what situations. As with an individual client, explain that once the desire for the first cigarette has been overcome, the desire for the others does not enter the picture. Ask all the members of the group to remember what went through their minds that morning when they had the first cigarette. Explain that not everyone may be able to do that. However, it is likely that some attendees will, and with those you can get them to change the submodalities of that signal.

Then you explain about ultradian rhythms, and about how people need to find a more useful way to punctuate the day than through smoking. Talk about the same concerns which people have in one-to-one therapy. Ask whether people smoke in order to change their mood, and educate them about stress management.

Phase 6: Teach attendees self-hypnosis

Here is a version of self-hypnosis more suited to groups than to individual therapy. It contains a few more elements and is designed to ensure that everyone enters a satisfactory state of inner focus and relaxation. Tell the group:

> "In a moment, we are going to do a simple technique called instant self-hypnosis. This is a way of putting yourself into a peaceful, calm, resourceful state any time you want. You won't need to be a slave to random impulses any more. You can use it to programme your own mind to plan your own future.

> "Now, everyone, look up at me."

Establish eye contact with each attendee in turn, then look directly in front of you.

> "I'd like you to be aware of your breathing. Building up a nice, natural rhythm of deep, easy breathing. Breathing from the diaphragm, just below your lungs, where your abdomen is. That's right. Filling the lungs with air from the bottom to the top. And every time you breathe out, can you expel all the air from your lungs, so that you're getting a really good air circulation? Just let your eyes close any time you want. That's right. And every time you breathe in, keeping your eyes closed, roll your eyeballs upwards, as if you were looking at the Third Eye in the middle of your forehead. Every time you breathe out, lower and relax those eyes, so that you're moving those eyeballs up and down with each breath. That's right. And every time you breathe out, say the word 'calm' to yourself, silently and mentally. And every time you breathe out, see the word 'calm', written right in front of you. And you can let those eyes lower and relax now, and let that quality of relaxation flow all the way down from your eyes through every muscle in your body. And every time you do this, you'll be putting yourself into a peaceful, calm, comfortable state.

> "Just be aware now of your conscious thoughts – that endless running commentary and picture show that we all have going on in our conscious awareness. You already know what it's like to watch TV. I'd like you to imagine that you're at home watching TV, on one of those old-fashioned TV sets in a dark wooden cabinet. That old TV set is situated at the other end of the room from where you are, so that its screen looks pretty small. Once you can see that TV, project your conscious thoughts onto that TV screen, so that you can now see those pictures in black and white and hear that running commentary on the TV set, while you stay sitting at the other end of the room. And then switch off that television set,

observe as the picture shrinks down to a white dot in the middle of the screen, and then disappears completely. And you can enjoy that. And if you can find twenty minutes a day to practise doing this, maybe first thing in the morning, during some break in the day, perhaps when you come home in the evening, or maybe last thing at night, then you'll be training your body in the habit of relaxation, which will have excellent long-term health benefits for you."

This metaphor helps many people to switch off the flow of conscious thoughts which can interfere with self-hypnosis. Keep a close eye on the participants and make sure that they are indeed relaxed. If you see someone's shoulders hunched up, for instance, then it is all right to place your hand on those shoulders and gently encourage the attendee to lower and relax them. The next stage in the group self-hypnosis is an exercise in substitution for smoking:

"You have a powerful imagination. And many times you have gazed at clouds in the sky at sunset, lit orange and pink and purple from the light of the setting sun. So as you continue breathing, in and out, in that endless rhythm of deep, easy breathing, just imagine that there is a small, beautiful, clear blue cloud right in front of you. Just inches away from your face. A cool blue cloud which contains wonderful healing, calming, invigorating properties. Gaze on that cloud in your imagination. And the next time you breathe in, breathe in some of that cloud – that cool, fresh, blue cloud. Inhale it deeply now, letting it into your body, down your throat, into your lungs. And hold it in those lungs for a couple of seconds. Feel that fresh blue healing, calming, invigorating cloud filling those lungs, flowing through the bloodstream, going to the brain, permeating your entire body just the way the smoke used to. And then exhale, expelling that cloud, and notice whether maybe the colour has changed. Inhale from that blue cloud again, hold that breath and feel that blue cloud refreshing, invigorating, healing, cleansing out the muck accumulated inside. And then exhale slowly and completely, seeing the changed colour. Breathe in from that cloud again – hold it – and breathe out again. In – hold – out. In – hold – out. And really notice the difference. (Pause.) And doesn't it give you at least as much satisfaction and pleasure as that other habit used to do? So you see how you can do precisely this same exercise of the imagination any time you want a moment to yourself, or to chill out, or to wind down. It really is that simple."

You then continue with the photo album metaphor, just as with individual therapy, which is presented here in the slightly different version suitable for group therapy.

"And as you continue to enjoy this experience of instant self-hypnosis, you can be aware that everything you experience is authentic, there's no right or wrong in any of this.

"And be aware now that in this very relaxed state, your unconscious mind has access to all of your memories, stored away in the back of your mind. Have you ever had that experience of rummaging through an old trunk in an attic filled with long-forgotten junk from way back when? And when you take out something and it brings back a flood of memories that your conscious mind had forgotten? Or how you can leaf through an old photo album and as you see those pictures, so many vivid experiences of people and places and situations flow into your conscious awareness?

"That's because all of your memories are stored away. Something like photographs in a pile of albums, stretching way back over the course of your life. Big blow-ups and small prints, colour pictures and black-and-white, digital prints and Polaroids, thousands of photos showing every moment throughout the course of your life. And your unconscious mind has full access to all those pictures, all those memories.

"And there was a time when you were a healthy, happy non-smoker. Maybe you did stop smoking for some weeks or months or years. Or even if you didn't, then there were all those years of your early life – your childhood, early teenage years, maybe even into young adulthood – when you were living as a healthy, happy non-smoker. Either way, I'd like you to take down that photo album which shows that wonderful time when you were living as a healthy, happy non-smoker. And find just one good day from that time. Maybe a day in which you achieved something worthwhile, or else just a day of relaxing and taking it easy. And have a good look at yourself on that really good day. Look at what you are doing. See the expression on your face. Notice the position of your body. Hear the things you are saying – and really notice the difference. And perhaps there's a piece of music that you find inspiring – and if so then you can play that music in the background as an accompaniment to that scene. And if you like what you can see and hear, then step inside your own body on that very good day. Feel the way your body feels. See what you can see with your own eyes. Hear what you can hear with your own ears, hear that inspiring music – and really notice the difference. And if there's any word or phrase which comes into your mind which can describe this experience, then you can say that word or phrase to yourself, silently and mentally, again and again. And as you do that, press your right thumb and your right forefinger together, forming a tight circle. And as you do that, silently and mentally say that word or phrase to yourself again and again. That's right."

In a group setting, it is easier to have the participants set up the anchor themselves. Here the anchor is formed by pressing the thumb and forefinger together to make a circle. Watch the participants to make sure that they are doing it correctly. If you have to help any of them, do so quickly and unobtrusively. Continue:

"Good. Now step out of that experience, loosen your thumb and finger and just clear your mind. What you've just done is set up an anchor. It's just the same as when you hear a piece of music that you haven't heard for many years, but it brings back a flood of memories of people and places from the time when that music was popular. Any time you want to bring back that experience, just press your right thumb and forefinger together and say that word or phrase, and it will come back to you.

"And now I'd like you to take down that photo album which shows your future life. Maybe you can open that album and have a good look at yourself on that date, or maybe it's all a bit obscure. But if you can, then open that album and have a good look at the photo of yourself one month in the future. [Name the date one month from now.] Look at the expression on your face. See what you're doing. Notice the position of your body. And really notice the difference. And if you like what you can see and hear, then maybe you can play that same inspiring music in the background as an accompaniment to this scene. And step inside your own body in that picture so that you can feel the way your body feels on [the date one month from now], see what you can see with your own eyes and hear what you can hear with your own ears. And really notice the difference. And then I'd like you to imagine that you are floating backwards through all the different photos which show everything that you've done in the past month, seeing it, hearing it and feeling it. And at an unconscious level, I'd like you to make all the different learnings and understandings that can make that future a reality in your life. And then I'd like you to float back, float back to [today's date], step inside your own body sitting in that chair and become awake and alert and refreshed, and allow your eyes to open."

It is probable that several members of the group will agree that they require a useful way of managing stress. If so, then include the technique of rapid variable stress management described in Chapter 6, before you awaken the participants. In the unlikely event that none of the attendees say that stress is an issue they need to deal with, then there is no need to include it.

Let the attendees take a few moments to come back to full waking awareness. Then ask them, "So, how did you find that little exercise?" Different people will have different experiences. Some will be able to vividly recall the memories you requested them to access, while others may have had difficulty in doing so. Remind the group that everything they experience is authentic for them as individuals, and that there is no right or wrong. Some people find it easy to visualise, whilst others make sense of the world more through feeling or sound. The one thing which everyone should have achieved is a sense of being more relaxed. Even if that is the only thing that they achieved from the exercise, they have still learned how they can make a change to the state they experience in the moment through a method more useful than smoking a cigarette.

Phase 7: Preparing for different situations in future

After teaching the participants instant self-hypnosis, then, just as with individual therapy, tell the group that there is no such thing as "just the one" cigarette, and that it is essential to know how to stay a non-smoker in every situation. Recommend the use of self-hypnosis particularly when facing the three situations where the temptation to smoke might arise: meeting an old friend who still smokes, getting through a difficult situation, and attending a social event at which people are smoking. Just as with individual clients, talk about the "moment of temptation" which might arise when a cigarette is offered, and how to deal with it by taking a decision just for that moment to gain the benefits which derive from being a non-smoker. Deal with the shift in energy and finding a positive outlet for all that energy. Deal also with the questions of weight control, alcohol, marijuana and socialising with smokers in the same way. Describe the nature of cravings and how to deal with them. Keep this phase of the event interactive, but make sure that it does not take up too much time or veer away from the main focus of the event.

Phase 8: The main group induction

Because you are dealing with a group of different individuals, you have to give them an induction which is going to be appropriate for most of the people most of the time. Here are several inductions suitable for groups. Whichever induction you choose, strike a balance between addressing the group as a whole and ensuring that each individual is going along with the process, at least to the extent of breathing slowly and deeply, relaxing the muscles and closing the eyes. The use of hypnotic music, which has been specially recorded for the purpose of assisting in trance induction, is recommended for any group induction (there is a discography in Appendix 4).

Whichever group induction you choose, at the start it is essential to get agreement from everybody to be hypnotised. You could say: "Ladies and gentlemen, it is now time for you to enter that creative part of your unconscious mind which will carry out that inner transformation which will enable you to live life as a non-smoker. You are about to experience hypnotic trance. If you are ready and willing to be hypnotised, nod your head." Make sure that everyone does nod their head. Then validate that by saying, "Good" or "Excellent".

Indirect "sleep" induction

The use of the word "sleep" to induce hypnotic trance is so well known that is has become a cliché, used in jest by many people when one first introduces oneself as a hypnotist. Therefore, I do not recommend that you use the direct command, "Sleep!", in any therapeutic context, individual or group, precisely for this reason. Nevertheless, in its origin, it was found that the use of this word in hypnotic inductions did produce a trance state which the unconscious mind entered as analogous to actual sleep – the hypnogogic state which we enter every night in those moments between being awake and being asleep. The purpose of this group induction is to gain the same effect by utilising the participants' experience of drifting towards sleep at night-time by the use of the clock.

After having gained agreement to be hypnotised, you say: "Now I'd like everyone to sit with your hands in your lap, and your palms turned upwards. And I wonder whether you've ever watched a beautiful sunset out in the countryside somewhere on a warm summer's evening, round about eight o'clock. Looking up at the vast sky, with clouds of orange and pink and purple. Shadows getting longer, and a cool evening breeze caressing your face. And on the horizon, the big orange-red sun just floating there, casting its colour across the sky and the landscape. While an antique clock somewhere in the distance chimes eight o'clock. And have you ever watched as that sun *v-e-r-y s-l-o-w-l-y* sinks below that horizon, little bit by little bit, so that more and more of it slips below the horizon while less and less of it is still above the horizon? As the clock strikes half past eight. And can you see that more easily with your *eyes closed*? Just let those *eyes close* any time they want, so that you can see only that beautiful sunset. Just watch that setting sun now as I pass along the group."

Go through the entire group, one by one, turning their palms downwards on their laps, and gently pushing the head downwards, in two easy movements, so that the subject assumes a foetal position, while you say the word "relaxed". If there are too many in the group to make this feasible, then tell them to do it themselves: "Now just carry out these two easy movements. First, turn your hands in. Second, gently push your head forward assuming a foetal position."

Continue with the following words, spoken with poetic rhythm:

Nine PM ... That sun sinks below the horizon, but its light still turns part of the sky mid-blue. Just sitting there, calm and relaxed.

Nine-thirty PM ... The whole sky dark, with thousands of bright stars visible. A sense of relaxation flowing down from the top of your head to the tips of your toes and fingers. Relaxed from the tips of your toes to the tips of your fingers.

Ten PM ... The moon rises and casts a pale white light over the landscape. With your *eyes closed*, let your imagination open. So that you imagine yourself sinking down into the darkness. [If anyone's eyes remain open, just quietly say to that individual, "Close your eyes."]

Ten-thirty PM ... Everything feels very heavy and tired.

Eleven PM … The whole of your body feels like lead. Your arms and legs feel like lead, so heavy and tired.

Midnight … From now on, no need to notice any of the sounds in the room. Noises just pass you by – like the rhythm of crickets, the rustle of the breeze, or the hooting of an owl at night. In fact, any sounds will send you deeper and more and more relaxed. Any sounds will send you deeper and deeper into this creative state of your imagination.

One AM … From now on, even just hearing my voice will send you deeper and deeper into your unconscious mind. In other words, deeper and deeper relaxed.

Two AM … From now on, with every deep easy breath you take, you will sink deeper and deeper into your creative inner world. You will feel more and more relaxed.

Three AM … And as you relax more and more with each hour of the clock, so you can find yourself descending into the world of your creative imagination, in which your unconscious mind is learning. In the meantime, you are going to be more and more relaxed, more and more heavy and tired, more and more drifting away.

Four AM … So that as you are consciously aware that your body feels more and more heavy, and more and more relaxed, so your unconscious mind is listening, active and learning. And it doesn't really matter whether your conscious mind hears my words or not, because it's the unconscious that I really want to speak to."

The one word which is not mentioned in the above is "sleep."

Elman-style authoritarian group induction
The following is an authoritarian induction in the tradition of Dave Elman. It is more likely to fulfil many people's expectations of what a group hypnosis session "should" be like. Here you are very much giving the orders and expecting obedience. It is particularly useful for a group which is used to obeying orders in an hierarchical institution, such as the armed forces, emergency services and many corporations. It is also recommended if members of the group have found it difficult to engage with the exercises earlier in the session which deal with internal realities (submodalities, self-hypnosis and so on).

Immediately after gaining the participants' agreement to be hypnotised, say to them:

"So sit straight upwards now, your back flush against the back of the chair, your feet flat on the floor and your hands in your lap not touching. Keep your eyes looking forward at me, and your attention on the sound of my voice.

"There is nothing on this earth – absolutely nothing – that can keep you from accessing the creative power of your unconscious mind and living the rest of your life as a healthy, happy non-smoker. Remember that you have chosen to enter this creative, powerful state of your unconscious mind for a specific benefit which is going to transform your health and your life for the better.

"So take a nice deep breath with me, and hold it. And release that breath. A deeper breath, and hold it. And release. And now the deepest breath of all; hold it. This time, as you release that breath, allow your eyes to close, listening to the sound of my voice. Shift the focus of your attention to that chair you are sitting on, be aware of how it supports you fully, so that you don't need to do anything but relax, and keep breathing slowly, deeply and evenly, from the diaphragm. That's right.

"Just allowing yourself to become more and more relaxed with each breath you exhale. Shift your attention now to your left elbow. Notice how that elbow rests comfortably. Maybe you become aware of your right hand, and notice the way it feels. Shift your attention towards the sole of your right foot. Just become aware of how the floor beneath completely supports it – and that drops you down deeper. And the deeper you go, the better, the more relaxed you feel with every breath you take.

"So now focus your attention on your eyelids. Relax those eyelids completely to the point where they will not open. You are in command. In a moment I'm going to have you test those eyelids; I don't want you to test them until you are certain that they will remain closed – just like locked garage doors.

"I want you to test those eyelids on the count of three. One, two, three. Good, stop testing, relax and let that feeling of relaxation flow through your entire body, from the top of your head, down to the tips of your toes. With each easy breath, allowing you to drop down deeper and then deeper. The deeper you go, the better you feel.

"And some of you are in a deep hypnotic trance already, while others are well on their way there. And in a moment I'm going to come along and pick up some of your arms, your left arm. That left arm should be loose, limp, relaxed. I know you could help me lift that arm, but don't. Let me do all the lifting today."

Move along the row and lift each left arm at the wrist to ensure that the arm is relaxed, commenting on each individual. "Excellent. Nice and limp. Good.

Wonderful." If anyone is insufficiently relaxed, then say to that person: "Deeper. No, looser, let it go, loose, limp and relaxed, good."

Return to the front of the group, and continue:

> "We achieve relaxation in two ways – mentally and physically. You're all doing superbly with the physical relaxation. Now it's time to relax mentally. Here is how we are going to do it.

> "In a moment, I will begin reciting the letters of the alphabet backwards from Z. It will be Z, Y, X and so on. Each time I say a letter, I'm going to say, 'deeper relaxed'. I want you to focus on the letter in your mind. You don't need to visualise the letter. This has nothing to do with visualisation; you just need to direct attention to the letter I say. Make that letter a burden that you want to get rid of, a burden you can get rid of by the time I get to Q or sooner, and as you do, notice how good you feel. Here we go.

> "Z, deeper relaxed, and the deeper you go … the more confident, the more secure you become, X, deeper relaxed … W, deeper relaxed … V, deeper relaxed … that's right … T, deeper relaxed, … Q, pushing all thoughts of all letters out of your mind and as you do, noticing how good it feels."

Note that in the above, the letters Y, U, S and R are omitted. What you are doing here is giving the subject's conscious mind a relatively difficult mental task, that of focusing on the letters of the alphabet in reverse order from Z. You are describing the letters as burdens that the subject wants to get rid of. You start from Z and then jump straight to X. By omitting Y, you have made the task even more difficult and confusing. Then you continue the sequence with W and V, but then jump straight to T, causing more confusion. Finally, you jump straight from T to Q, omitting the two letters S and R. The purpose is to create a context in which the subject's conscious mind simply abandons the mental task and enters a deep trance. Continue:

> "In a moment I'm going to count to three. When I get to three, not before, I want you all to be seated upright and open your eyes and look at my raised hand. I'm then going to say two words; those two words are 'sleep now', and I will snap my fingers.

> "This is your signal to return to this pleasant state of inner awareness you're experiencing now, allowing your eyes to close, and your body to go loose, limp and relaxed. Each and every time we do this it will drop you down twice as deep, so you can feel twice as good, twice as confident, twice as secure. One, two, three, sleep now (snapping your fingers), one, two, three, sleep now …. (Adopting a more assertive tone:) One, two, three, sleep now. One more time: one, two … three, sleep now.

"From this point forward, let your unconscious mind respond to everything you hear me say. Your conscious mind can go anywhere it wants, doesn't need to hear my words at all. Let that creativity, that protective force within you, carry out this wonderful transformation. So that everything that I say will instantly become your reality."

Yogic group induction

The following induction combines several concepts from yoga. Naturally, it is especially suited to groups where several members have had experience of yoga or other meditative techniques.

"Just sitting there, place your hands in your lap, those hands cupped as if ready to accept the inner flow of the life energy of the universe.

"Yoga means awareness. And you can shift your awareness. Just by *closing your eyes right now*, you can switch off the external visual field and see instead that mass of colours inside your eyelids that corresponds to nothing in your internal world. Be aware of the internal world of your body now – the sound and feeling of your breathing, your pulse and heartbeat, how the different parts of the body are so different in their levels of relaxation and warmth.

"Yoga means union – union with the universe. Yoga teaches about the life energy of the universe – prana it is called. Just imagine that prana now, perhaps as a shiny white flow of healing energy. As you breathe in, so you are breathing in that prana, letting it fill your body and mind and spirit. And then breathing it out, long and slow, in an endless rhythm. Breathe the prana in – and out, in – and out. Focusing on that moment between the breaths, that moment when there is no breath.

"So be aware now of the sounds in this room – the music, my voice, your own breathing, the hum of the projector, that clicking of the radiators. And the sounds outside this room: the traffic somewhere, birds singing, kids playing, the rustle of the wind. [Of course, you refer to whatever actual sounds are audible.] Sounds never disappear completely. So extend your awareness further to the sounds beyond – to voices, music, machines, nature, the ocean and so much more. Can you hear them? Maybe as a distant undifferentiated murmur perhaps, or maybe as distinct sounds. It doesn't really matter.

"Just be aware of what you can see. With your inner eye, that is. Even with your eyes closed, you can remember what this room looks like. And can you imagine floating upwards, out of your own body, so that you are looking down from the ceiling at your own body sitting there? And can you imagine seeing that body becoming more and more limp, relaxed and comfortable by the moment? The breathing *s-l-o-w-i-n-g d-o-w-n*, in a very healthy, pleasant way. The muscles loosening more and more. The face very still because its muscles are so relaxed.

Losing track of time, and of space. Mind wandering freely, the conscious mind, that is, while the unconscious mind is listening and learning and making sense of everything in its own way. And you can just watch that body from this distant point. As if you were a body without a mind, a mind without a body.

"Just be aware of what that body feels. The temperature in the air. That endless rhythm of the breath. The pressure of the chair on the back. The comfort in the muscles. The levels of relaxation in different parts of the body. The temperature in different places. And you can make changes to the experience of that body. Increase the distance between the left shoulder and the right shoulder. Increase the distance between the head and the feet. That's right. Just noticing how easy it is to change that awareness. Yoga knows of no limitations of time or space – awareness can shift inside or outside – to the past or the future – it's all under your direction.

"And as you continue breathing in the life energy of the universe like that, in and out, in and out, focus your attention now to that space inside your head, that area of darkness behind your eyes. The yogis teach that there is a Third Eye in the middle of the forehead, in between our two ordinary eyes. Just imagine that Third Eye now as a triangular window through which you can breathe, in and out, in and out. And as you breathe in through that triangle – deeply, slowly, evenly – direct the flow of that prana to that space behind your eyes, cooling it, calming it, cleansing it. Breathing it in cool – and noticing how warm it is when you breathe out. Noticing that moment in between the breaths, when there is no breath.

"And in yoga the centre of the body, just below the navel, is the *hara*. Put your thumb in your navel, and go inwards from the palm of your hand to the centre of your body. The very centre of your being – which spreads that energy through thousands of small channels throughout your psychic nervous system. So breathe that prana into that centre of your being in the centre of your belly now. Feel it glowing with energy and power and enjoy the sensations of comfort, ease, satisfaction and fulfilment. Peace inside me; peace to my right; peace to my left; peace below me; peace above me; I am peace.

"And let that peace spread from the *hara*, through every part of you. Just imagine that psychic nervous system as a complex network of blue waterways – rivers, streams, canals, waterfalls, channelling that feeling of peace throughout every part of you, from the top of your head to your fingers and toes and everywhere in between.

"Just imagine that in the little stream on the little finger of your right hand is a little boat. And inside that boat is a pile of candles. Big candles and small candles. Candles of different colours. Thin and thick and round and square candles. Candles scented with different perfumes. So just take out a small candle and place it there in the little finger of your right hand. So that its light illuminates the inside of that little finger. Is it a flickering light or a steady light? And once you can see that candlelight and feel its warm energy, take that boat down that blue waterway into the middle of your right hand and place another candle there, so that that hand, too, is illuminated in the same way. And then place a candle in each of the other fingers of the right hand – and the thumb. And then take that little boat up the channel of the right arm and into the torso and place candles all the way throughout your entire body. Different sizes and shapes and colours and scents of candles for different parts of the body, so that more and more of your body is illuminated by those candles on those rivers, streams and canals. Placing those candles everywhere across your torso, up through your neck and every part of your head, down your left arm to the left hand and fingers, down your stomach, down your hips, down your left leg and foot and toes, and down your right leg and foot and toes. So that those candles, big and small, different shapes and sizes and colours and scents, are illuminating every part of your body.

"And just imagine that your skin becomes transparent, so that you can actually see that blazing illumination of those candles throughout that complex of beautiful blue waterways that flow through every part of your body. Just experience that for a moment.

"And then know that your body, mind and spirit are merely an inlet connected through the breath to that vast ocean of prana in the universe. So that as you continue to breathe in and out, in and out, in that endless rhythm, so you are continuously fuelling that illumination in your body from the infinite energy of the universe.

"Yoga means union. Union with the universe. So let your awareness spread now, out of your own body, beyond the confines of this room, following the sounds outside to spread above and beyond this building, beyond this whole street, this whole town, this whole country, and beyond to this continent, and this planet. And beyond that to this solar system, this galaxy and the entire universe.

"And while your awareness continues to be absorbed in that experience of union, so your unconscious mind is listening, and open and learning. And it really doesn't matter whether your conscious mind hears my words or not, because it's the unconscious, creative imagination that I want to speak to."

Image-based progressive relaxation induction
This version of the progressive relaxation induction is suitable for groups. Instead of relying on the subject passively accepting suggestions to relax different parts of the body, it gets the subject actively involved by drawing on experiences which affect the state of the body.

"As you sit there, listening to the sound of my voice, perhaps you can shift your awareness to how the different parts of your body feel. Notice the softness of the fabric at those points where your clothing touches your body. Notice the pressure of your shoes on the floor – and is the left shoe or the right shoe the more comfortable of the shoes? Notice the temperature in the air, and how different parts of the skin have different levels of coolness and warmth. And how different parts of the body have different levels of relaxation, too. And as you focus your awareness inside your body now, which one of your hands feels most relaxed now? The left hand or the right hand? Whichever it is, how do you know that that hand is the most relaxed one? Can you identify the feeling that tells you that it's the most relaxed? Can you even see a colour, a light, an energy that you can associate with pleasant relaxation? Can you let that feeling, colour, light, energy, flow through that hand so that you know what it's like for a part of your body to be really very relaxed indeed? And perhaps you can transfer that sense of relaxation to the other hand, too, that they are both just as relaxed. And if you *close your eyes*, you can see that energy and light so much more easily.

"And the next step is to breathe that relaxation all the way through your body. So breathe deeply, slowly and evenly, filling the lungs with air from the bottom to the top. And exhale, building up a rhythm of deep easy breathing. And as you do so, draw that relaxation from those hands up the length of your arms, so that you can see and feel that same sensation flowing through those arms. Continue breathing, every breath sucking that sensation of relaxation through the shoulders, up the neck and through the head, down the chest, down the stomach, through the hips and down the legs, right down to the feet and toes. So that the whole of your body becomes just as relaxed as those hands.

"And be aware now of the temperature at the different points in your body. And what's the temperature in the hands? Can you imagine placing those hands onto a patch of bright sunlight on a table? Or on top of a wall under a baking sun in mid-summer? Or cupping a mug of tea or coffee in your hands? Or putting on a pair of oven gloves, opening the stove and lifting out a delicious-smelling, bubbling casserole dish. Or wearing a snug, comfortable pair of thermal gloves on a winter's day. And how do those hands feel now? If they feel just a little bit warmer, then you already know how easy it is to change the way you feel without having to make any great conscious effort about anything.

"So that you can enjoy imagining what it would be like to have a huge jug full of hot massage oil made for you, just the way you like it. Hot oil, for relaxing, warming and healing. Just see that hot oil in that jug on an open fire in front of you. And there are jars containing herbs and spices and flavourings and leaves and essences of different substances with different delicious scents. And you can lift out a pinch of the ones you like the look of and the smell of and drop them into that jug and give it a good stir. So that it's pleasantly warm and smells nice. Just test it by putting in your thumb and forefinger and feeling its warmth, softness and quality, the way it feels on the skin, the temperature just right. Notice how it actually permeates through the skin to the thumb and finger beneath.

"And now that jug of hot, scented oil is raised above your head. And it's being poured gently onto the top of your head. And remarkably, this oil flows down through the top of your head into the interior of your skull. So that that hot oil flows down through the muscles inside your head, around the scalp and down the face, loosening and melting those muscles, so that your forehead, eyes, cheeks and chin are saturated with the warm, pleasant flow of that scented oil. Flowing through the muscles of the jaw, so that those jaw muscles relax completely and maybe your jaw drops. That's right.

"While the flow of that hot oil slowly descends down your neck and across your shoulders, melting away tension as it permeates those muscles with its warmth and healing. Flowing down your back, dripping down through every bone in the spine, loosening and easing those muscles as it sinks downward. And down your arms, too, that hot oil cascading down through the muscles and bones of those arms, melting and softening them. That hot oil easing down the chest, too, spreading through all those ribs and the muscles around them, flowing down the stomach so that all that tension just dissipates as that oil descends through it.

"That wonderful warm, scented oil, dropping down deep inside you, and now through your hips, and getting caught up in the inner circulation of your system. So that that healing oil spreads through the areas of stress and tension and cleanses them, clearing out hot debris, so that it rises again through the circulation, warmer and carrying that debris with it as it circulates back upward, leaving behind a clean, refreshed, tranquil interior of your body.

"While fresh warm oil flows down inside both hips, loosening and cleansing all those muscles, flowing down the bones into your legs, and all the way down those legs, relaxing, easing, comforting and healing, down to your feet and toes. And beyond those feet and toes, draining all the excess tension and toxins as it sinks deep into the ground through those feet and toes. And through the arms, hands and fingertips, too, the oil flowing down to the floor and beneath that floor, removing the debris and leaving behind freshness and warmth and health and vigour.

"That hot scented oil continuing to flow all the way down your skin, outside and inside, so that you might find that any concerns or upsets which had been on your mind are themselves being melted and drained away, so that you simply experience the moment in the moment. So that it really doesn't matter how long you enjoy this for. Even time can be melted away. And your conscious mind can keep enjoying this flow of melting and relaxing, while your unconscious mind is listening, learning and making sense of my words in its own way."

Phase 9: The message to get across in trance

In a group session, you want to include as many elements as possible. Some techniques will connect better than others with different participants. Therefore the following message to be got across in a group session contains elements from both the main session for individuals and the follow-up. Again, the goal is to get across the general ideas rather than the exact wording. It is also important to add any issues which are of particular concern to one or more participants.

Using the group mind for smoking cessation

"And as you sit there, listening to the sound of my voice, and becoming more and more relaxed with each breath you take in – and out, in – and out, just reflect now on everything you've already learned here about how to live as a non-smoker. And reflect on the fact that so many individuals are present here today in a group united for that one common purpose. And reflect on the energy, the power, the strength which is generated by the presence of a group of people united in a common experience for a common cause. And the group is stronger than the individual. Every individual here has already decided, consciously, to become a non-smoker. And most of you are well on the way to making that a reality. But there are still a couple of people here who are wrestling inside. Sure, they understand the benefits of becoming a non-smoker, but there's still a part of them clinging to the habit. A part of them that's questioning the whole process of becoming a non-smoker. And that's just fine. Many people who have experienced just those thoughts have walked out of here and lived as non-smokers permanently. In order to make certain that that happens with every single individual in this room, we are going to tap into the power of the group mind. Since before the dawn of history, communities have tapped into the group mind, the collective unconscious, in order to achieve healing. That's what we're going to do right here and right now. In a moment, I'm going to come along and tap every second one of you on the shoulder. Those whom I tap on the shoulder will be the sender."

Move swiftly from left to right along the length of the group, tapping every second person on the left shoulder. Make sure that you tap the shoulder of the person sitting at the right-hand end of the semi-circle, even if it means skipping the person on their left. Continue:

"If I did not tap you on the shoulder, you are the receiver. Now, sender, keeping your eyes closed, I want you to think about the person sitting to your left. You know what that person looks like. That person, like you, is here to become a non-smoker. I know that you want that person to successfully achieve that goal. Receiver, just sit there, passively, being open to receiving whatever pops into your awareness. There's no right or wrong in this – whatever you experience is authentic. Sender, I want you to see and hear and feel what that person's daily life will be like as a non-smoker. Just get an impression of what that is going to be like. And I want you to make an affirmation for that person: "You are a happy, healthy non-smoker." Say that affirmation in your own voice and project it onto that impression of your neighbour as a non-smoker. Continue to hear that affirmation in an endless rhythm. And then get in touch with the healing energy of the universe, however you imagine that. It doesn't matter what your beliefs are – just direct that healing energy towards that impression with that affirmation. And then, on the count of three, when I say the word 'send', in your mind, I want you to send, project, throw, or flip that impression, affirmation and energy, onto your neighbour on your left. So that it falls onto your neighbour and envelops them like a cloak. Nod your head if you understand. (Each sender nods.) Good. One, two, three – send. (Pause.)

"Good. Now I want everyone to swap roles. Those who just sent, you are now receivers. Those who just received, you are senders. Senders, focus your attention on the person sitting on your right …"

You then repeat the above process with the roles reversed. After that, continue:

"Good. And now you are all going to be both senders and receivers. I want you to build up that healing energy and feel it flowing through you. I want you to see an impression of every member of this group becoming a non-smoker right here in your mind's eye. Say that affirmation: 'You are a healthy, happy non-smoker.' On the count of three, I want you to project that energy, that impression, that affirmation, across the entire group, and at the same time open yourself to receive that same energy, impression and affirmation from everybody else. Just take ten seconds to do that on the count of three. One, two, three – send! (Pause for ten seconds.) Excellent."

This technique both makes use of group dynamics and helps to bypass the critical faculty. Many people attending a smoking cessation group event understand the benefits of stopping smoking intellectually, but part of them wants to cling to the habit, so they keep mental reservations. Some will "hide in the crowd" and rationalise along the lines that, "The other people here may well stop smoking, and good luck to them, but I don't think it'll work with me." Here you are utilising that attitude. Each attendee uses their benevolence towards the others to "send" the attitude conducive to becoming a non-smoker to their neighbour, and also passively "receives" the same attitude, in both cases without mental reservation. In order to do that, each attendee has to create within their mind an internal representation of the resources required to become a non-smoker, both by "sending" it and "receiving" it. It really doesn't matter whether the attendee – or the hypnotherapist – believes intellectually in the reality of a "group mind" or not. What matters is the drawing out of unconscious resources which this technique carries out.

Learning set and deepening
We now move towards more familiar hypnotherapeutic techniques. This section includes the learning set and deepening.

"And ever since the day you were born, your unconscious mind has been helping you to learn, helping you to adapt successfully to new situations.

"When you learned to eat with a spoon, can you remember how difficult that might have seemed? Sitting in the high chair, how awkward it was to hold it? How you kept missing your mouth? How that food kept falling out of the spoon? Until little by little, you learned how to handle that spoon, so that you could eat from it without spilling. And later on you learned how to use a fork and a knife, and maybe chopsticks, too. That's because your unconscious mind enabled you to master the use of cutlery, so that you can enjoy a meal without consciously having to think about how to hold or move the cutlery at all.

"And when you first learned to tell the time, can you remember learning about the long hand and the short hand, and how if the long hand was pointing to the 12, and the short hand was pointing to the four, that it meant it was four o'clock. And if the long hand was pointing to the nine and the short hand was in between the ten and eleven, that meant it was a quarter to eleven. Pretty soon you could look at a clock or a watch and in an instant you'd know the time without having to consciously think about the hands or the numbers. Even one of those ultra-modern clocks with only the hands and no numbers or marks – one glance and you know the time. Your unconscious helps you tell the time.

"And later on, as you grew up, in exactly the same way, your unconscious mind enabled you to learn about life, about people, about yourself. Your unconscious always protects you and looks after you as best it can. And your unconscious mind is helping you to learn again today, helping you to learn something of great benefit to you, your health and your future.

"And just as your unconscious has helped you to learn so many things, so too, throughout the course of your life, your unconscious mind has left stuff back in the past which is no longer relevant to what's important to you now. When you were a young child, you were probably very interested in toys and fairy stories and kids' cartoons and the tooth fairy. You probably enjoyed making sandcastles and eating jelly. Later on, when you became a teenager, you forgot all that young kids' stuff. As a teenager, you wanted to prove yourself, become part of the gang, come across as cool and glamorous and sophisticated. Some people start smoking as teenagers, others as young adults. But however you started, that earlier version of yourself focused on living in the moment. At that time in your life, you were ready to try anything, to do anything. You had no knowledge of long-term health issues, or what was really important in life. And that's when the habit of smoking started. Later on, you learned more about life, about people, about yourself. As an adult, you learned to deal with people in a more grown-up, mature and responsible way. You took more responsibility, took a long-term view of what was important. Maybe you built a career. And maybe you took on responsibility for other people, too, in various ways. In so many ways, you've left back in the past the teenage way of blowing tantrums, showing off, bunking off from things. Because that earlier version of yourself who took up that habit of smoking doesn't really exist any more. That person is back in the past, and now you're taking charge of your own life, your own health, and your own body, and you're not willing to risk that life, that health, that body for anyone, least of all that youngster who still had so much to learn about what's really important in life. As an adult, as a grown-up, you're choosing to take responsibility for your life, your health and your body, and you're going to leave back in the past that habit which that earlier version of yourself took up, back in the past where you left jelly, sandcastles and all those other childhood and teenage things."

Deepening and a "room of health"
The deepening used here includes a combination of the metaphor of a staircase, numbers and the colours of the rainbow. The "room of health" is a metaphor for unconscious learning. Continue:

"And as you continue to allow that group energy to resonate through every part of you, perhaps melting away any reservations or doubts that may have been there, so you can imagine yourself at the top of a grand staircase. And stretching below you are seven broad steps, which will take you deeper and deeper, until you face a door at the bottom of those stairs. Each of those seven steps is lit with a different colour, each colour of the rainbow, as if sunlight is coming through a skylight separated into sections tinted with different colours. So that as you walk down that staircase, so you are bathed in the light of one colour after another. And with every step you take downwards, so your muscles loosen more and more, and you may find your mind wandering, as you become deeper and deeper relaxed. So ready – step one – red – bathed in red light. Down to step two – orange, permeated with orange sunlight. Step three – bright yellow light. Four – green – saturated in green light. Five – blue – awash in blue light. Six – purple – covered in purple light. Seven – white – bathed in pure white light. Facing the door now, as you step through that door you will be in that place where real learning takes place.

"And inside that room, you find yourself in a beautiful chamber, exquisitely furnished and finely decorated just the way you like it, with so many fine items which you like so much. But no ashtrays. Looking out through large windows on a lovely sunlit stretch of hillside leading down to the banks of a river. This is your room of health. A room of comfort and ease where you have everything you could possibly want. Excellent health, long life, high energy, a clear skin, a sense of freedom and independence. A non-smoker. In this room you have all the habits that are consistent with your excellent health and none of the habits which in the past used to harm your health. In this room, your unconscious mind turns your decisions into reality. And any time you want to return to this room, just say the words "room of health" and you'll find yourself right back here.

Direct suggestions to stop smoking

"And I want to speak to your unconscious mind about something of great significance – to you, your health and your future.

"You have already decided to become a non-smoker. And here in this room of health, because it is your wish, your decision, to become a non-smoker, it becomes your reality. Now and forever. You have broken free from the smoking habit for the whole of your future life. It really is as easy as that. And you can take pleasure in the fact that you are now a non-smoker.

"And when you first took up that habit of smoking, can you remember your body resisting? Perhaps you were coughing, feeling dizzy, wanting to be sick, even turning green. That's because your body was resisting that poison. The only way your body can communicate with you is through its physiological reactions, and when you were feeling sick, your body was saying, 'Stop it. That smoke is a poison, I don't want that smoke. Reject it. Stay a non-smoker.' But you forced your body to accept that smoking habit. And later on, when you wanted to quit smoking, maybe you found it difficult to quit, because your body didn't realise that you were quitting. But today, in this very relaxed state, in which your decision to become a non-smoker is becoming a reality, your unconscious mind now understands that you are now a non-smoker, and that fact, that understanding, can permeate every part of you, so that your body welcomes this breathing space that you are giving it, now that you are achieving freedom from the smoking habit.

"And can you remember how good it was for all those years of your early life when you lived as a healthy, happy non-smoker? As a young child, as a teenager, how you lived life and never once even thought about smoking. And can you remember that one good day during that non-smoking life that you experienced? I'd like to ask the unconscious part of your mind to bring back that experience now, so that once again you can live life as the non-smoker you were as a child and a young teenager. And now you know all about self-hypnosis, how to create that relaxed, comfortable, resourceful state any time you want it, and how to be prepared for any and every situation, so that you stay a non-smoker in all situations. So that you will remain a non-smoker for ever and ever.

"So it really is that simple. You know that you're a non-smoker – so you don't smoke. You will never smoke tobacco again in any format. So that you don't smoke a cigarette or a cigar or a pipe or a roll-up containing tobacco. And if someone offers you a cigarette, all you have to say is, 'No thanks, I don't smoke,' and whenever you say that, your unconscious mind will welcome the fact that you are now a non-smoker. So you go through your daily life, and you find the whole focus of your attention shifting to the worthwhile, beneficial things all around you, focusing your thoughts on what's really important to you, so that you forget about that old habit. Smoking for you is in the past, behind you. It all happened a long time ago. Just as you've moved forward, from being a young child, to being a teenager, to becoming an adult, and as you've left so much stuff back in the past as you've progressed, and changed the whole focus of your attention in so many areas to what's really important in life, so also you leave that old smoking habit in the past where it belongs, in the same place where you've left eating jelly and playing with toys and so much else."

Telling a story
The rest of the message to the group is contained within the frame of a "story" about a previous group, talking about different individuals in that group and what they experienced.

"And just so that your unconscious mind knows how to make sure that you stay a non-smoker in every situation, I'd like to tell you a story about a really excellent group, just like this one, who came here to become non-smokers just a few months ago. They were from different walks of life, male and female, and different age groups. They had all been smoking for a long time. Some of them had actually quit the habit for some time – one of them for three weeks, another for six months, yet another for five years. Another one kept quitting for about four days at a time but kept going back to it. Some of them hadn't quit since the day they started. But they all had some things in common. All of them were non-smokers for six or eight hours every night when they were asleep. And most of them surprised themselves when they went on a long-haul flight to Australia or Thailand or India or some such place, that they could stay on that plane for eighteen or twenty-four hours and the fact that they didn't smoke simply never bothered them. And when they visited someone's house who they knew were non-smokers, they were happy enough being non-smokers. And others could go all day at work and not even think about smoking. So already there were situations were they could enjoy life, be themselves and be entirely happy being non-smokers. And every one of them was sick to the back teeth with smoking and wanted to just escape from that habit. And every one of them was a creative individual whose unconscious mind had to find its own way towards the new and healthier lifestyle.

"So those who had already successfully stopped smoking at some time in the past, whether for weeks or months or years, were able to remember just how they did it. Some had quit through willpower, others through patches or gums or Zyban, still others through a moment of insight and internal transformation. There was one lady who had quit smoking as soon as she learned she was pregnant. One gentleman stopped when he moved into his new house. In that very relaxed, focused state of inner awareness, they were able to go back to that moment of success and repeat it. The body already had the memory of that transformation. So I asked the unconscious mind to repeat that success. And that's exactly what happened. I asked them to look into a photo album showing that time when they successfully became non-smokers. They looked through that album and saw pictures of themselves waking up in the morning feeling fresh, breathing fresh, clean air into strong, healthy lungs. Feeling high energy flowing through mind and body. In those photos, their skin looked fresh, young, and clear, their teeth white and clean. Those pictures showed how they were able to enjoy family life, working life, social life, travelling, dealing successfully with unexpected setbacks, and staying non-smokers. And enjoying that life for day after day, week after week, month after month and for some of them, year after year. Then I asked them to go back to the photo at the beginning of that album, so that they could see that moment when they did become non-smokers. Whether it was through willpower, or patches, or gums, or Zyban, or acupuncture, or hypnosis, or through group therapy, or from reading the book by Allen Carr, just that single moment of transformation – that breakthrough, that epiphany, when that individual became a non-smoker. I asked them to look at that picture of themselves in that moment, notice the expression, the bodily posture, in that moment of transformation. Then I asked them to step inside that body and feel the way they felt in that moment, repeating that epiphany, that breakthrough, that transformation. And it happened again just as easily as it had before. And because they knew all about self-hypnosis, and how to prepare themselves for every situation out there in the real world, they were able to stay non-smokers for ever and ever.

"And for those in that group who had not stopped smoking since they smoked their first cigarette, I asked them to look through that photo album which showed their early years – as children, as teenagers, in some cases as young adults, in which they lived, year after year, never once even thinking about smoking. I asked them to look at one good day from those years, and really notice the difference. And I asked their unconscious minds to find the way to repeat that success, to make the conscious desire to live as a non-smoker into a living reality. To leave that habit back in the past where it belongs. A temporary decision in a temporary situation which no longer had any relevance to them.

"And it really was that simple. They went out there and they lived daily life as non-smokers. Their bodies made the most of that breathing space they gave it, and expelled all the tar from the lungs, the carbon monoxide from the bloodstream, and the nicotine from the entire body. They felt their energy level rise, as their heartbeat and pulse went down to their proper level. Their senses of smell and taste came back, so that they could appreciate the fresh, clean smell in their clothes, their home and their fingers. Their bodies' natural defence mechanisms came back. They had no desire to smoke when they woke up, during breakfast, or when they went outside. And when they were travelling, they simply forgot about that old habit. At work, too, they were non-smokers. Socialising, enjoying hobbies and sports and family life – they had no desire to smoke. They learned to practise self-hypnosis and gain control over their experience in the moment. One guy found that he could handle stress so much more easily that way. Another learned to get more pleasure out of less alcohol, so that he could enjoy socialising with smokers and non-smokers alike. One lady learned to get in touch with her body's natural hunger, and eat the foods that body needed, so that she actually lost weight when she quit smoking. Most people found the whole process smooth and easy once they learned to manage their experience in the moment. However, one lady did still experience cravings for the first few days after the session. But she knew that those cravings only lasted for ten seconds, so all she needed to do was distract her attention for ten seconds and they would disappear. She would check her emails, drink a glass of water, eat an apple, and that craving simply disappeared. And as her body cleansed itself and became a non-smoker's body in those two weeks after the session, so too those cravings disappeared. And those people in that group who were parents took pleasure in the fact that they were setting such a great example to their children, that those children became far more likely to grow up as non-smokers now that their parents were themselves non-smokers.

"And you – every one of you in this room can do the same thing as those members of that other group."

"Three key ideas"
At this point, if time permits, you can add the "three key ideas" technique used in individual therapy. Continue:

"I'd like your unconscious mind, too, to learn and recognise that you no longer want to smoke. So that you can take on board these suggestions, learn them just as you've already learned to walk, to run, to read, to write, to drive and so many other things that you have already learned to do at an unconscious level. So that that desire to smoke first thing in the morning has simply disappeared. And you can enjoy that taste of your early-morning hot drink so much better now that that film of tar has disappeared from the top of your tongue. No desire to smoke when you are at home, when you go outside, while you are travelling, or during your daily routine. Now that you know all about ultradian rhythms and self-hypnosis, you can move yourself up and down that numerical scale to find just the right level of alertness and relaxation for every working situation. And as a non-smoker, your concentration improves, your reflexes get faster and your concentration improves, so that you will achieve more and easier and better in your career, or whatever you do in life, now that you are a non-smoker. You have no desire for tobacco after lunch or dinner, and by eating like a gourmet, giving your body the water-rich foods it really needs, you will become or remain just as slim as you want to be. And when you are partying, socialising, drinking and dining, you enjoy being a non-smoker – whether it be with friends, family, colleagues, clients, people you know well or people you've only just met. And you can trust your body to protect you from other people's poisonous smoke. And if anyone offers you a cigarette, you simply say, 'No thanks, I don't smoke.' You simply let the conversation move on, and pretty soon you forget about that moment.

"And it's as easy as that. You go through day-to-day life and find yourself focusing on what's really important to you – so that bit by bit you forget about that old habit. It all happened a long time ago and the memory of it becomes hazy and vague. And if a stray thought about that old habit passes through your mind for a moment, as a non-smoker you can simply let it pass through like so many other stray and random thoughts. No point in struggling with that stray thought – you will focus on something more useful and valuable. So you forget about the whole thing, certain that you are and will always be a non-smoker.

"Indeed, any time you find yourself reflecting or daydreaming or contemplating this transformation, you think of how much your life has improved now that you are a non-smoker. Just think now about those three benefits that you wrote down on that sheet of paper when you walked in here. See and hear and feel yourself enjoying those benefits as I count. One … two … three … (Pause.) Thinking about how good it is to wake up in the morning, feeling fresh, breathing fresh, clean air into strong, clean and healthy lungs – with high energy flowing through mind and body. You think about how good it is to enjoy much better health, to know that you've greatly extended your life, greatly improved your long-term health prospects. Looking in the mirror and seeing your skin fresh, young, healthy, energised, your teeth clean and white and shiny. How good it is to have your senses of smell and taste come back to their proper level, so that you can enjoy the fresh, clean smell on your fingers, in your hair, on your clothes, in your home. Thinking about all the extra money that is now yours, and the worthwhile, beneficial things you can spend that extra money on, things that will improve the quality of your life. Thinking about the social freedoms you now enjoy, how you can now go anywhere you like, do anything you want, and enjoy that experience. How happy those people are who mean so much to you, now that you've made this transformation to excellent health and long life. You think of the excellent example you're setting to those whom you influence. And you think of that sense of independence, knowing that you are free, moving forward to a healthy future life of freedom.

"And day by day, week by week, month by month, as you become more and more used to life as a non-smoker, so your mind will become more and more clear and calm, while your body becomes more and more supple and relaxed. Finding your energy level rising as all that trapped physical and mental energy comes back at your disposal. So that you find it easier to live life resourcefully – drawing on the power you already possess within yourself to deal more effectively with the world, with the people you deal with, with every situation. Cultivating the habit of self-hypnosis, finding the most appropriate level of alertness and relaxation for every situation. Finding yourself enjoying life more, taking life in your stride, opening yourself up to those things that the unconscious really wants for you deep down. And as you leave that old unwanted habit back in the past where it belongs, so you find yourself positively embracing this better and healthier future.

"And I'd like you to take down now that photo album which shows your future life. And have a look at the photo of yourself one month in the future – [name the day one month from now]. Notice the expression on your face, the way you hold your body, hear the things you are saying, and the things you can hear, and really notice the difference. And if you like what you can see and hear, then step inside your own body in that picture, so that you can feel the way your body feels, see the things you can see, and hear what you can hear, and really notice the difference. And I'd like to ask your unconscious mind to take just three silent minutes to find the best, the most powerful way to make this future a reality in your life. Three silent minutes to reflect on everything you've experienced, everything I've said, three silent minutes to make it happen – starting now."

Three silent minutes follow. Continue playing the music during those three minutes. Then:

"And this process of learning, understanding and transformation can continue today, tonight, tomorrow and in the days ahead. And I know that you are wondering … and it is a good thing to wonder … because … that means … you are learning many things … And all the things … all the things … that you can learn … can bring you new insights … and new understandings … And you can, can you not?

"So now that your unconscious mind has learned how to carry out this wonderful transformation in your life, I'm going to wake you. I will count from seven to one, and you will wake up just a little bit with each number. Until on the count of three, your eyes will open, and by the count of one you will be completely awake. Every part of you will be back in the here and now, except that part of you that used to smoke, and you will awaken feeling great, optimistic, alert and energised, with a sense of achievement flowing through every part of you. So ready: seven, waking up, six, coming back to the here and now, five, waking up, four, waking up, coming back to the here and now, three, opening your eyes, two, one, wide awake, wide awake."

Wait until everyone – or almost everyone – is fully roused. When they are, move directly on to the closing group ritual.

Closing group ritual

The moment immediately after the subjects have been aroused from trance is a very powerful one for rapid and effective techniques. The participants are still in a state in which the unconscious is active and learning, and the critical voice of the conscious mind, with its sceptical running commentary on everything, has not yet come back. This closing group ritual utilises this powerful moment and at the same time draws on group dynamics and the concept of affirmation to seal in each participant's transformation. Once everyone's eyes are open, say:

"Now everybody raise your right hand like this, as if making the scouting oath."

Raise your own right hand as if making that gesture. Once everyone's hand is raised, continue:

"Everybody repeat out loud after me: 'I am a non-smoker.'"

If necessary, gesture with your left hand to ensure that every attendee says the same words, more or less in unison. Continue:

"From this day forth," – attendees repeat – "I give my body health, energy and long life." Attendees repeat. "I commit to success in living as a non-smoker." Attendees repeat. "I successfully deal with every situation as a non-smoker." Attendees repeat. "And I shall never …" – attendees repeat – "ever" – attendees repeat – "no matter what" – attendees repeat – "smoke any cigarette," – attendees repeat – "cigar" – attendees repeat – "roll-up" – attendees repeat – "pipe" – attendees repeat – "snuff" – attendees repeat – "hookah" – attendees repeat – "the exhaust pipe of a car with its engine running" – "a factory chimney belching out industrial waste" – "or any other source of carbon monoxide, nicotine and tar" – attendees repeat – "in any form whatsoever" – attendees repeat – "from this day forth" – attendees repeat – "for the rest of my life" – attendees repeat.

Although the above passage is framed in negatives, note that each negative is followed by another which is more unlikely and bizarre. The purpose of the above passage is to change the subjects' internal representation of smoking. You are leading the subjects into forming an unconscious association between forms of smoking which they have previously considered "normal" (cigarettes, cigars and roll-ups), less familiar and somewhat eccentric forms of consuming nicotine (pipes, snuff and hookahs), and absurd and ludicrous forms of smoking (a car's exhaust pipe and a factory chimney). Finally comes a reminder that all the items just mentioned are sources of carbon monoxide, nicotine and tar. The goal is to form a chain of associations so that the concept of smoking a cigarette is perceived to be just as unpleasant, ludicrous and poisonous as smoking a car's exhaust pipe or a factory chimney, and therefore just as repugnant. The participatory state of emotional arousal and collective affirmation, combined with the subjects' motivation and the effect of the techniques they have already experienced in the session, justifies the use of a "negative" approach in this particular case.

You can say the above with tone and expression that are so exaggerated that they come across as way over the top. While the participants might take your style as being somewhat tongue-in-cheek, the very process of making this affirmation in such a context attaches great importance to it at an unconscious level. Allow some thirty seconds of silence at the end of this ritual.

Checking your work

Then you address the one attendee whom you think has responded best out of the group. Choose someone who has both found it easy to access and change internal representations in the early exercises, and who has successfully entered a deep trance. The external signs of trance include: stillness of the facial muscles, lightening of the skin, slow, deep and even breathing from the diaphragm, slower pulse (visible at the neck and sometimes at the wrist and leg), unconscious movements (most commonly of the head), and rapid eye movement (visible under the eyelids).

Ask that person how they feel now. Assuming that that individual says something positive, it will tend to have a good effect on the other participants. (This is, of course, precisely why you pick the person whom you think has responded best.) Then ask the others, in turn, about how they feel. Go in approximate order from the one who has responded best down to the one who has responded least well. If one or more people think they need further help, then take this opportunity to do rapid work with them. For instance, if someone says that they feel a craving for a cigarette, get that person to change the submodalities of that feeling and diffuse that experience. If a person says that they are attending a party that evening, and are worried about the prospect of being offered a cigarette, then repeat the "moment of temptation" technique, showing that individual how to gain control over momentary thoughts and therefore stay a non-smoker. By so doing, you are demonstrating to the whole group that they are not mere passive recipients of hypnotic messages, but are resourceful individuals with the power to make rapid changes to subjective experience in the moment and therefore take control over their own destiny.

Then you can say, "Many congratulations, everybody. You are now non-smokers. Give yourselves a round of applause." Let them applaud.

Then you talk about their future lives as non-smokers. It is a good idea to finish by doing the emergency stop (described in Chapter 9). Of course, the difference in a group setting is that you get each attendee to touch a point on their own wrist rather than you touching it.

Finally: "That's about it for this evening. Remember, any time you feel you'd like to return to one of these events, you are most welcome. And if anyone wants to have a word with me privately and in confidence about anything, I'll be here to help you in any way I can." Of course, you answer any questions or give any advice to anyone who needs it. If you have products for sale and sign-ups for self-hypnosis classes available at the back of the room, this can bring you increased revenue.

Your goal is to keep promoting these group seminars, build a reputation for good results and build long-term income. Try to arrange the events at the same place on the same night of the month (for instance, every last Thursday of the month). Any person who has paid once should be entitled to come back as many times as they like. Apart from the fact that you are giving the person what they need to stop smoking and stay stopped, it looks good if there are many in attendance rather than a few.

Chapter 14

Smoking cessation for the corporate market

After having gained significant experience in achieving good results with one-to-one smoking cessation, and, preferably, in running smoking cessation groups open to the public, the hypnotherapist is in a position to offer smoking cessation seminars to the corporate market. This is where the hypnotherapist goes into a particular company and runs a training event at which those of the company's smoking employees who choose to quit the habit can do so.

Recent changes in legislation have prohibited smoking in all workplaces in the United Kingdom. In May 2006, laws passed by the Scottish Parliament to that effect came into force north of the border. The Health Act 2006, passed by the UK Parliament, imposed the same smoking ban on workplaces in Wales and Northern Ireland in April 2007, and in England in July of the same year.

This new legal situation creates a potential problem for those companies which have hitherto allowed employees to smoke somewhere on their premises. Many organisations have allocated a smoking room where smokers can take their breaks. Other firms, particularly in the leisure, catering and hospitality sectors of the economy, have permitted smoking by both employees and customers. These companies now have a strong need for smoking cessation services in order to enable them to adapt to this new legislative environment. (See Appendix 1 for more information about these laws.)

If you are a hypnotherapist who can enable companies to meet this challenge by running smoking cessation events for employees, you are therefore meeting a specific corporate need. In order to do that, it is necessary to know something about the role of corporate training in the business world. It is necessary to educate corporate decision-makers about the service, convince them of its value, and provide evidence of its effectiveness. Once the corporate client requests the seminar, it must be delivered smoothly and effectively, in a way the participants can understand, and must "do what it says on the tin" – that is, the attendees should actually stop smoking and stay stopped permanently. It is also vital to provide back-up support afterwards in the form of further seminars, telephone and e-mail support, and, if necessary, one-to-one therapy, for any employee who needs it.

Piloting

Before you approach the corporate market, I recommend that you do at least three pilot sessions. A pilot session enables you to gain experience with groups. These could be either smoking cessation seminars open to the public, which people pay as individuals to attend, or free smoking cessation seminars which you offer to the staff of an organisation such as a hospital or registered charity. By organising and delivering these pilot sessions, you will pick up numerous small but important details which are difficult to learn from a book but which will make your group seminars much smoother, more fun and more effective. Plan the first such seminar down to the last detail. When the event takes place, it is advisable to video it with a camcorder, with the permission of attendees, and view it later. Make sure that all the practicalities are handled smoothly. If anything came across as clumsy at any point, make a note of it and get it right the next time. Notice which techniques in the session connected powerfully with attendees, and which need to be worked on in order to ensure that the next group finds them easy. Improve your handling of those techniques for future group sessions. Also, give attendees a feedback form with questions about their experience and their evaluation of the event, and encourage them to fill it in and return it anonymously. Read the comments and make any changes warranted by them. Follow up the attendees, with their permission, and ensure that they have indeed stopped smoking.

Then repeat the process with a second group seminar, using a sharpened approach developed as a result of your experience. Once you are satisfied, from the feedback from the second event and the camcorder footage of it, and the results from the follow-up, that you have got the formula right, run a third pilot group session using that refined formula. Once you are satisfied with the results from the third seminar, you are ready to approach the corporate market.

Approaching the corporate marketplace

Once you have gained experience in enabling smokers to quit the habit in your group seminars, you have a valuable service to offer those companies which are seeking a smoke-free workforce. Your task is now to ensure that company deci-sion-makers know what you have to offer and how it can help them achieve that goal. You need to justify the cost of the seminar and convince those deci-sion-makers to commit to ordering your seminars.

From the hypnotherapist's point of view, the advantage of approaching the cor-porate market is that it helps to overcome one of the central problems of hypno-therapy. The quicker and more effective hypnotherapists are at helping clients in one-to-one therapy, the faster they lose their clientèle. They mostly have to find new individual clients whom they have not previously helped. The same is true of public group smoking cessation seminars: those attendees who become non-smokers by attending such an event have no need to return to another. By contrast, once you are regularly providing smoking cessation services to a large company, it is likely that they will have many existing employees who want to become non-smokers, and will continue to require your services in the long term as new smoking employees join the firm. Also, it becomes possible to provide the same corporate client with seminars for employees about such topics as stress management, public speaking, motivation and communication with NLP. This greatly reduces the effort involved in acquiring new clients, and can bring in significantly increased continuous revenue.

However, do be aware of the potential downsides of approaching the corporate world. It is likely to take a long-term, sustained effort, possibly over several years, to reach corporate decision-makers and become established in the field. It is likely that you will have to adapt – at least to some extent – to the corporate culture. It means communicating in their terms and fitting into their system. You will find yourself dealing with a lot more paperwork and bureaucracy than when working with individual clients. Also, bear in mind that companies rarely pay for training immediately after it takes place. You will mostly have to invoice them, and sometimes it can take months of persistent reminders to have those invoices settled. This could lead to cash-flow problems if you have paid for an outside venue, such as a hotel or conference centre, where the training has taken place. In the rare cases where a company becomes insolvent before having settled your bill, then as a creditor you are unlikely to be paid at all.

If, having accepted these realities, you decide to approach the corporate market, then it is important to focus your efforts in the most efficient way. Think in terms of specialising by both geographical area and economic sector, at least at the start.

Obtain a map of your area on the Internet with your home at the centre. Draw a circle with a twenty-mile radius around that central point. (If you live in a low-population area such as the Scottish Highlands, make it a fifty-mile radius.) Make this the area in which you will direct your initial efforts. In choosing the companies to approach within that circle, focus on those in the field in which you worked before you became a hypnotherapist. If you used to work in construction, for instance, obtain a list of building companies and their suppliers, such as equipment retailers and specialist employment agencies. If you worked in hospitality and leisure, collect details of hotels, restaurants, bars and venues such as snooker halls and bookmakers'. Your experience in the particular industry enables you to "speak the language" of decision-makers in these companies. Because you know about the specific challenges faced by employees in that industry, your seminars will be more relevant and useful for them.

Now your goal is to ensure that each company on your list knows that you offer corporate smoking cessation seminars. It is essential to have a website, even if it is only a single page with a brief description of what you offer and your contact details. A website is rarely enough on its own to convince a potential corporate client to choose your services, but it is necessary to have one to establish credibility in the corporate world. Write letters to each company on your list, describing your earlier experience in that industry, and how you now offer smoking cessation seminars which can help the company comply with current legislation. Offer to visit the company and explain about your seminars and how they can help that firm's employees.

Join at least one local business networking group, and offer to speak at meetings of local organisations of which corporate decision-makers are members. Examples include the Chamber of Commerce and service clubs such as Rotary International. Send a news release about your service to local newspapers, radio and television stations and business periodicals. Keep copies of any coverage you obtain. Write articles for business magazines, newsletters of organisations, and websites. Again, keep a portfolio of these to show potential clients in order to build credibility. Make sure that your talks and articles contain information which is useful to your audience even if they do not immediately avail themselves of your services. Your goal is to come across as – and indeed to be – a valuable local institution to whom businesses can turn when they need to achieve a smoke-free workforce. Take a long-term view of your corporate services. When you meet business decision-makers, make it your goal to educate them rather than subject them to high-pressure selling. Let them know that you will be there to help them at any time in the future they require your services.

Whatever results you obtain with your marketing efforts, persist with them. If you get little or no response from the first companies you approach, contact others within your area, including those in different industries. If you do get a good response, you still need to maintain your marketing efforts to ensure that other potential clients know what you have to offer. Keep talking to local groups, writing for business publications and sending out sales letters and news releases.

Make sure that you are ready to provide your corporate seminars at short notice, if necessary. Smaller companies tend to be dominated by one overall boss who can take decisions instantly. If such an employer approaches you at the end of a talk at a service club, and requests a seminar for next Wednesday afternoon, make sure that you are fully set up to provide it. Decisions in larger companies tend to involve several individuals and take longer.

Ensure also that you have public liability insurance specifically for training. Corporate clients are likely to request a copy of your insurance certificate when they order your services.

The role of training in the corporate world

The hypnotherapist who intends to provide smoking cessation seminars to the business world needs to understand the overall context within which corporate training operates. The training function, of which smoking cessation is part, must be in harmony with the organisation's structure, and must be seen to contribute to the organisation's success. The effectiveness of any organisation is the extent to which it achieves its objectives. Everyone in the organisation must be focused on those objectives, and the role of training is to assist in the achievement of those same objectives.

Human resources development (HRD) is defined as the integrated use of training development, organisational development and career development to improve individual, group and organisation effectiveness. Within HRD, corporate training focuses on the learning process that achieves more effective performance. Performance itself is defined as the outcomes, results, accomplishments and achievements of individuals. The effectiveness of performance is assessed by examining the content of an action (what), the way it is executed (how), the result of an action (effect), and the quality of that result (how good). Business decision-makers insist that corporate training must contribute to effective performance if they are to fund it. The "logic of training" is that the organisation benefits, in terms of increased production, greater quality and reduced costs, when improvements in competence are manifested in job performance. Managers will expect a corporate smoking cessation seminar to achieve these results.

Following the model of management expert Tom Boydell, director of the consultancy Inter-Logics, corporations divide training needs into three types: *organisational*, *occupational* and *individual*. Within each of these three categories, training needs are divided into two sub-categories:

(1) training needs *generated by* change, such as new products, technology, and laws, and
(2) training needs which must be met in order to *produce* change; for example, to increase productivity, improve morale and change the corporate culture.

Before the Health Act 2006 became law, the purpose of corporate smoking cessation seminars was in most cases to *produce* change: the company took an internal decision that it was desirable to have a non-smoking workforce. Now that workplace smoking is illegal, such seminars are more generally understood as training *generated* by change – in this case, by the impact of the legislation. Thus the new laws have led to a change in companies' perception of the benefits of smoking cessation at the organisational, occupational and individual levels.

The funding of corporate smoking cessation

A key question in corporate smoking cessation is how it is to be funded. The funding of an employee's attendance at your seminar will take one of three forms.

With **company funding**, the company pays the whole cost. If the management is convinced that enabling an employee to quit smoking will benefit the business, and not just the employee as an individual, then it is more likely to choose company funding. This could be the case in, for example, the leisure, entertainment and hospitality industries, where smoking by staff had been accepted before the workplace smoking ban, but where there is now a need for corporate culture to change in order to comply with the new laws. With company funding, there is more likely to be a high take-up, as employees are being given the opportunity to quit smoking and gain the approval of management at no financial cost to themselves.

With **voluntary (employee) funding**, the employee pays the cost of attending. With voluntary funding, it is important to keep the cost of attendance per head low in order to encourage widespread participation.

Joint funding is a combination of company funding and voluntary funding, and can be in any proportion, such as 75 percent paid by the company and 25 percent by the employee. The advantage of this is that it can make it affordable for the employee to take part, while retaining a strong incentive for success, as the employee is likely to be motivated to get value for money.

If a company considers smoking cessation to be primarily a benefit for the employee, rather than an objective for the company as a whole, it can still offer participation in a smoking cessation seminar as a staff benefit. Successful companies recognise the need for a contented workforce, and seek to expand the range of staff benefits they offer in order to attract new employees and retain existing ones. If a company offers participation in a smoking cessation seminar as an employee benefit, it can be made available in one of three forms:

(1) **a company-funded benefit** – paid for by the organisation
(2) **a flexible benefit** – a "menu" of company-funded benefits, from which the employees can choose
(3) **a voluntary benefit** – organised by the company but paid for by the employees themselves.

Designing the corporate smoking cessation seminar

In a larger company, the management will typically want to determine whether a smoking cessation seminar fits the learning needs of employees who want to quit smoking, and whether it is likely to be cost-effective. It does this through an internal process known as a training needs assessment or training needs analysis (TNA).

Once the company's managers have accepted the idea of a smoking cessation seminar, recommend that they distribute a brief written notice via e-mail to all employees explaining what the seminar is all about and encouraging those employees who want to quit smoking to volunteer to take part in it. If you can arrange that this notice includes a message from senior management which encourages participation, and perhaps emphasises the enhanced career opportunities that employees will enjoy after they quit smoking, this may convince some who still have reservations about becoming non-smokers.

However, attendance must be voluntary for it to be effective. Make sure that the notice encourages employees to ask you any questions they might have, in confidence, without obligation, and without undue pressure to volunteer. Then, when everybody who wishes to do so has signed up, the trainer meets again with the managers to fix the most convenient date and location (from the company's point of view) to hold the smoking cessation seminar. Because it is certain that both managers and employees will be busy with their jobs, it may be necessary for the trainer to be courteously persistent in ensuring that each stage in this process is completed.

Every corporate training event has to pass the three Es test: it should be *effective* (achieve what it sets out to do), *enjoyable* (from the attendees' point of view) and *efficient/economical* (worth the time and cost). In order to achieve this, you will need to adapt the smoking cessation seminar to the particular group with which you are working. For example, the kind of music you play in the background should be appropriate for the people in the group. If you are working with a group of senior partners in an accountancy firm, the ideal introductory music would be Baroque masters such as Bach and Händel. With employees of a nightclub, all of whom are under 25, modern ambient music would be more appropriate. My own view is that it is best to build rapport at the start of the event by playing the sort of music that would be likely to be enjoyed by those attending. By making an educated guess as to the sort of music they would like, you are pacing them by playing music that it is assumed they are comfortable and familiar with. You can then gradually lead them through the process of becoming a non-smoker, an idea that they might be less comfortable with at the beginning of the seminar. Later in the event, when you induce the main trance, you could play less familiar music. My preference is for the CD *Astral Journey* by Dick and Tara Sutphen. This both helps to induce trance and to encourage attendees to think differently by mismatching their usual way of doing things.

In choosing which techniques to include, consider the attendees' likely model of the world. Accountants might do better with descriptions of neuro-linguistic programming and metaphors which draw on their familiarity with the detail-oriented process of auditing accounts. For instance, you could talk about a spreadsheet, in which changes to one number in a cell can lead to big changes to many other numbers, due to the complex formulae which link them. By analogy, a small change to an individual's experience, such as changing the submodalities which cause them to smoke, can enable them to become and stay a non-smoker and enjoy all the health, career, financial and social benefits which are linked to that. With the young nightclub employees, you could include dramatic demonstrations of hypnotic phenomena and techniques of "group consciousness" which might come across as silly or improbable to the accountants.

Do as much advance research as reasonably possible to find out about the daily working routine of your participants, so that you can tailor your approach to the realities they experience on the job. With the accountants, you are likely to focus particularly on stress management; nightclub workers might be more interested in how they can remain non-smokers in an environment of high alcohol consumption. If you are providing seminars for an industry in which you worked previously, you will already know a great deal about what people in that field need. If you are approaching a sector in which you have not actually worked, then research the working routines of employees in that sector and then approach many companies in that sector with a view to providing your seminars. For instance, under the Health Act 2006, smoking in a commercial vehicle used by two or more employees is now illegal. If you want to provide smoking cessation seminars for the road haulage industry, you could research the challenges faced by lorry drivers, and develop techniques specifically for them to handle long drives while remaining non-smokers. You can then approach all the haulage companies in your region and offer them smoking cessation seminars which include these particularly relevant techniques. If a company in a sector you have little knowledge about calls you and requests a seminar, then you can ask them what specific issues their employees need to address in becoming non-smokers, and do as much other research as time allows before the event to tailor your seminar to that company.

Capture and maintain the interest of the particular group by relating as much as possible to their business. If you are providing smoking cessation services for a company involved with sport, such as a fitness centre, golf course or sports equipment retailer, then teach the group how to use submodalities, cognitive self-talk and self-hypnosis by explaining that just as successful sports performers train and practise in order to stay at their peak, so too the participants can practise these techniques in order to remain permanent non-smokers. Explain the nature of trance by saying:

"Some of the most outstanding sporting heroes have experienced this sense of detachment from conscious awareness during their greatest moments of achievement. They feel as if a force outside of them has taken them over and enabled them to surpass themselves. The great footballer Pelé, who gave an inspired performance for Brazil in the 1955 World Cup, later recalled that 'he played that whole game in a kind of trance'. And Dr Roger Bannister, the first athlete to run the four-minute mile, said afterwards that from the half-way stage he had a feeling of 'complete *detachment*'. David Hemery broke the world record in the 400 metre hurdles, and won by the widest margin in the history of the Olympics. He later said that he had no need to force his legs to work; it was as if his unconscious mind was controlling them. Arnold Palmer claimed that there was 'something spiritual, almost spectral', about certain rounds of golf. 'I'd liken it to a sense of reverie – not a dreamlike state, but the somehow insulated state of a great musician in a great performance'; the musician is aware of what he is doing, on such occasions, but his playing is dictated 'with an internal sense of rightness – it is not merely mechanical, it is not only spiritual; it is something of both, on a different plane and a more remote one.'[1]

"What we're going to do in a few moments is induce that same powerful creative state in everybody here in this room. Everyone here has that same potential to become a champion deep inside. Many successful winners in the sporting world cultivate and work on the inner game of tennis, or golf, or running, or what have you. We're going to work on your inner game of health and life and success and bring out that potential so that all of you become non-smokers. And each of you will win the gold medal of longer life, excellent long-term health, greater fitness, improved career prospects and saving thousands of pounds a year. So everybody put your feet flat on the floor and focus on your breathing ..."

Sports enthusiasts are fascinated to hear about these true experiences. Any attendees who may have been sceptical about hypnosis before the event will find themselves drawn in and inspired by these anecdotes. If you tell the stories above with enough intensity, the critical faculty of the attendees' conscious minds are bypassed even before you have formally induced trance.

When you are commissioned to do a smoking cessation seminar for workers in a particular occupation or industry, research the literature about the psychological aspects of that industry and drop in a few anecdotes. With salespeople, you could talk about the psychological techniques used in the layout of retail stores in order to encourage sales by appeals to the customer's unconscious. With information technology staff, you could describe how NLP breaks down the structure of subjective experience into series of subroutines which can be reprogrammed for improved results. The more you present your seminar so that it makes sense to the participants, the more effective, enjoyable and efficient it will be for them.

In designing your corporate smoking cessation event, if the organisation expects corporate trainers to use PowerPoint slides, then match their expectations. Adapt your slides for each organisation by putting the client's corporate logo on the bottom left hand corner of the master slide, and adding or changing slides to ensure that they are as relevant as possible to the specific group. Using PowerPoint ensures that the main point that you want to get across is visible. Visual aids also maintain a high level of energy in the room.

Preparing for the training event

Before running the seminar, prepare your materials according to the particular group with whom you will be working. You will probably need to produce a written training plan. In the corporate environment, everything of significance is documented. The corporation will need documents for its records. The session plan (also known as a lesson plan) is a written description of what you intend to happen, in the required sequence, and acts as a reminder. A session plan for a smoking cessation seminar might be as follows:

Session plan

Course title: Smoking cessation

Code: [the client may provide this]

Prepared by: [your name]

Date: [seminar date]

Learning objectives: To enable the attendees to stop smoking and know how to stay non-smokers in every situation.

Target audience: Smoking employees who want to quit the habit and have chosen to attend.

Maximum class size: 12   **Minimum class size:** 2

Essential prior knowledge: None

Learner preparation: None

Learner materials: Initial form, CD, written handout of techniques, multiple-choice test, feedback form, certificate

Equipment: Overhead projector (supplied by venue), PowerPoint slides, CD player with CDs, posters and Blutack (all supplied by trainer)

Duration: Three and a half hours (approximately)

Evaluation/validation: By participants on feedback form at end of event, by management after the event. Evaluation of attendees by trainer should take the form of a later follow-up to enquire whether the attendees have indeed stopped smoking.

Comments: In the event of relapse to smoking by one or more attendees, a subsequent seminar will be organised which they can attend.

Schedule

Prepare a schedule specifying what is going to happen and when. This document both informs the management as to what their employees will be taught and enables the trainer to stay on track and cover everything without exceeding the allotted time. In practice, the actual course of the event will probably deviate somewhat from the schedule, depending on the needs of the specific group and how many questions they have. The trainer may even omit certain stages or include material not written in the schedule, should it be deemed appropriate to the attendees' needs. The fact that the schedule is written down enables such flexibility without the risk of veering too far off track or overrunning the allotted time. Of course, the schedule can easily be revised for future seminars.

The best time of day for a corporate smoking cessation seminar is the afternoon, so that it ends just at the time the employees would normally finish their working day. This enables them to focus on the event without worrying about tasks they have to get back to, and also gives you the morning to thoroughly check everything and arrive in good time. The best location to hold the event is the company's own premises. However, if the company does not have a suitable vacant room, or if, for instance, a suitable room is too noisy, it may be necessary for the trainer to book a room at a local hotel or conference centre. The disadvantages of the latter are that attendees have the added task of travelling to and finding the venue, and that substantial costs are added to the whole project, which the corporate client will have to pay in addition to the fee for the training.

Course title: Smoking cessation

Time	Session	Objectives	Method	Materials
2.00pm	Welcome and introduction	Build rapport and future pace a successful result	Greet each attendee on arrival. Music playing, posters on walls	Introductory forms, pens, CD and player, PowerPoint slides
2.05pm	Discussion of how people start smoking	Provide understanding of the smoking habit and the workings of the unconscious	Recollections of attendees, explanation by trainer	PowerPoint slide
2.15pm	Discussion of previous smoking cessation	Find out who has stopped smoking before and educate attendees about importance of staying stopped	Recollections of attendees, explanation by trainer	PowerPoint slide
2.30pm	Gaining control over immediate experience	Teach attendees how to gain control over experience through NLP submodalities	Asking about current smoking experience, accessing memories of the impulse to smoke and changing them	PowerPoint slide
2.50pm	Self-hypnosis	Teach attendees self-hypnosis	Use instant self-hypnosis, observe participants, discuss experiences afterwards	PowerPoint slide, CD and player
3.15pm	Staying a non-smoker in all situations	Teach attendees how to stay non-smokers with cognitive self-talk, visualisation and affirmation	Discuss the situations to be prepared for and show how to use techniques	PowerPoint slide
3.30pm	Tea break			No smoking!
3.45pm	Workplace stress management	Teach attendees about the nature of stress and how to control it	Ask about attendees' experience with stress and teach them stress management	PowerPoint slide
4.10pm	The issues of weight, socialising and alcohol	Teach methods of successfully dealing with these issues as non-smokers	Ask about concerns regarding these issues. Teach methods of dealing with any issues the attendees mention	PowerPoint slide

Time	Session	Objectives	Method	Materials
4.25pm	Energy and cravings	Teach attendees to handle increased energy and deal with any cravings	Ask attendees about their recollections regarding energy levels and cravings when they quit previously. Teach methods of dealing with them	PowerPoint slide
4.35pm	Open discussion	Deal with any issues specific to one or more attendees	Invite attendees to raise any personal issues, and teach ways of dealing with them	PowerPoint slide
4.45pm	Trance induction	Induce trance in attendees in order to achieve unconscious learning to become non-smokers	Explain the creative nature of hypnotic trance, induce it and make powerful suggestions to become non-smokers	PowerPoint slide, CD and player
5.10pm	Last-minute issues		Deal with any issues arising after awakening	PowerPoint slide
5.15pm	Certificates, questionnaires, feedback forms and handouts	Test attendees' knowledge of what they have been taught and gain feedback. Give study materials to enable them to stay non-smokers after the session	Ask attendees to fill in multiple-choice questionnaire and feedback forms. Give CDs, written handouts and certificates	Questionnaire sheets, feedback forms, pens, CDs, written handouts, certificates
5.25pm	Benediction	Give attendees a message of encouragement and self-belief	Emphasise each person's resourcefulness	None
5.30pm	End of seminar			

In delivering group smoking cessation seminars, the trainer must be in a peak state. Therefore, wherever the event is being held, allow plenty of time to get there, so that you arrive early and unrushed. Use the extra time to make sure that everything that you need from the venue's management is in place at least half an hour before the start time of the event. Once you have set everything up in the room, use self-hypnosis to put yourself into a state of maximum resourcefulness immediately before the seminar begins. Just before the seminar, stand erect and imagine that your head is holding up the sky. Imagine that a hook on the crown of your head is being pulled upwards by a crane. Then maintain that posture as closely as possible throughout the event. The provider of corporate training can never afford the luxury of an off-day; it is essential to get it right first time, every time. John Grinder, the co-founder of NLP, was once asked what the most useful things are for a trainer to pay attention to. He replied, "First, pay attention to your own state. Second, pay attention to your own state. And third, pay attention to your audience's state."[2]

Unless the company specifically asks for it, do not make a video recording of a corporate event. (This is distinct from your early group events when you are learning how to do it). The presence of a camcorder raises privacy issues, and in any case will tend to make participants more self-conscious. If the company's management does request that a video be made, then ensure that the signed consent of each attendee is obtained before recording begins.

During the seminar, project enthusiasm and repeatedly establish eye contact with each participant. Keep your head and body as still as possible throughout as this makes it easier for attendees to keep their attention on you. When you do need to walk from one spot to another, make those movements swift, bold and purposeful, and keep them to a minimum. Keep your non-verbal communication congruent with your words. Finish each word and sentence, and avoid verbal pauses.

Before the event, check with the company's staff that your computer is compatible with their equipment. IBM-compatible PCs using Windows predominate in the corporate world. However, Apple Macintosh is widely used in creative industries such as advertising and design. If you have an Apple Macintosh, it is theoretically supposed to be compatible with Windows. However, the reverse is not true: if you use Windows and they have a Mac, they will not be compatible. In such a situation, you could either print the slides out on transparencies and place them on an overhead projector, or use the flipchart. Make sure you know in advance what the technical set-up will be.

If you are not using your own projector, make sure that you know how to use the organisation's projection equipment system. Run through all your slides beforehand to ensure that you have everything set up and ready. Switch the projector off when it is not in use. Do not leave a slide on the screen after you have moved on to the next point. Do not leave white light on the screen, as this is uncomfortable for participants' eyes.

At the end of the event, give each attendee a written handout and a self-hypnosis CD similar to those you give your individual clients, a questionnaire, a feedback form and a personalised certificate which you have signed.

The evaluation process

The process of evaluation is central to the provision of training in the corporate world. The management will assess the overall value of your training, the attendees will assess you as a trainer, and you will assess the participants in their response to your training. Evaluation enables corporate leaders to "prove" the connection between investment in training and an improvement in organisational performance. Evaluation:

- can be used to justify expenditure on future programmes.
- makes it possible to compare the effectiveness of different approaches.
- enables improvements to be made on the next occasion.
- records learning achievements and motivates learners.
- indicates to what extent the training's objectives have been met, and whether it has been cost-effective.

The most common model of assessment is the management expert Donald L. Kirkpatrick's concept of the four levels of evaluation[3]. According to a survey by the American Society for Training and Development, it is used by 67 percent of organisations in the United States. The four original levels are:

(1) **Reaction.** What did the participants think of the programme?
(2) **Learning.** Were the learning objectives met in terms of skills, knowledge and attitudes learned?
(3) **Behaviour.** To what extent can a change in job performance be attributed to the programme?
(4) **Results.** What are the effects on the organisation or department of the changes in behaviour in terms of cost savings, quality improvements and output increases?

Jack Phillips, another management expert, added a fifth level to Kirkpatrick's model:

(5) **Return on investment** (ROI). What are the deeper financial implications? This involves carrying out a cost-benefit analysis, leading to a cash value for the training.

More recently, a sixth level of evaluation has been added:

(6) **Intangible benefits.** This is applied where the data is too difficult or expensive to connect to monetary values, or where the management is satisfied with intangible data. An example would be a noticeable increase in employee satisfaction after the training.

The evaluation of a corporate smoking cessation seminar would be likely to go through the following with regard to the above stages:

(1) **Reaction.** The management may require feedback forms from the employees. They might provide the forms themselves. If not, you can provide your own.

(2) **Learning.** Assessment of what the attendees have learned can take the form of a multiple-choice questionnaire (see below).

(3) **Behaviour.** The management will assess whether each person who attended the smoking cessation seminar has in fact stopped smoking and stayed stopped.

(4) **Results.** Beyond determining whether employees have become non-smokers, the management will want to assess how far this has led to greater efficiency and productivity, and reduced absenteeism.

(5) **Return on investment.** The management will want to calculate how much money has been saved by a more productive workforce, the elimination of any fines for illegal smoking, reduced fire risk, lower insurance premiums and health care costs, and the longer working life of experienced employees, in proportion to the cost of the training.

(6) **Intangible benefits.** This could include higher workforce morale and appreciation by employees for the provision of the smoking cessation seminar. It could include better corporate image and identity, contribution to corporate social responsibility, and part of a positive assessment by a quality programme such as Investors in People (IiP).

We will now look at how you can fulfil the trainer's part of the evaluation process.

1. Reaction

Write an assessment of each attendee and how you feel they responded to the event. Remember that it is the therapist's responsibility to ensure that the techniques make sense to the participants, so make sure that everyone understands and can master the techniques. In addition, it is likely that the management will want each seminar attendee to complete an assessment form about you as the trainer. It could be that they will provide their own such assessment form. If they ask you to provide it, then set it out as follows:

Training assessment sheet

Name of attendee:

Name of trainer: [your name]

Attendee's job title:

Course title: Smoking cessation

Code: [company supplied]

Location of training:

Date of course:

General assessment	Answer	Comments
Did you choose to attend this course?	Yes/No	
Did you identify your learning objectives beforehand?	Yes/No	
Did you discuss these with your manager?	Yes/No	
Were your objectives met? In other words, have you become a non-smoker?	Yes/No	
Should the design of the course and its materials be changed?	Yes/No	
Overall, was the trainer competent?	Yes/No	
Overall, are you satisfied with the course?	Yes/No	
Please add any further comments you would like to make.		

Specific assessment	Answer	Comments
Did the trainer introduce the event well?	Yes/No	
Was the trainer effective in educating you about smoking and how people stop?	Yes/No	
Do you feel that you are able to gain control over your immediate experience through self-hypnosis, submodalities, visualisation and cognitive self-talk as a result of the training?	Yes/No	
Do you feel that you can manage stress more effectively as a result of the training?	Yes/No	
Do you feel that you are well prepared with regard to socialising, drinking, solving problems and staying slim as a result of the training?	Yes/No	
Do you feel that you know how to handle any cravings as a result of this training?	Yes/No	
Do you feel that you became a non-smoker as a result of this training?	Yes/No	

General assessment	Answer	Comments
Would you recommend that other employees who want to become non-smokers sign up for similar future trainings?	Yes/No	
Overall, how would you rate this training? (Please tick one answer.) ❑ Highly satisfied ❑ Satisfied ❑ Moderately satisfied ❑ Neither satisfied nor dissatisfied ❑ Moderately dissatisfied ❑ Dissatisfied ❑ Highly dissatisfied		
Please add any comments you may have. 		

2. Learning

At the end of the seminar, give each attendee a multiple-choice questionnaire about the material taught on the course. The purpose of the questionnaire is partly to remind the attendee of what they have just learned, partly for the trainer to be certain that each attendee has absorbed the necessary knowledge, and partly so that the company management can see what has been done. Make sure that this is both short (no more than ten questions) and so simple that everybody will get it right. It is not a final degree exam. The questionnaire might go as follows:

Questionnaire

Name of participant: _____

Please answer the following questions by placing a tick after the correct answer:

1. If I experience an impulse to smoke first thing in the morning, what is a useful way of changing that impulse?

    (a) Identify the submodalities of that impulse (such as size, location, colour and sound), and make changes to them with my conscious mind.

    (b) Say to myself, "I definitely don't want to smoke a cigarette."

    (c) Stay in bed until the impulse goes away.

2. What is a good way to induce self-hypnosis for relaxation?

    (a) Make my muscles tense and breathe quickly from the upper chest.

    (b) Play Baroque music on a CD player, close my eyes, breathe slowly, deeply and evenly from the diaphragm, expel all the air from the lungs, silently say the word "calm" and imagine seeing the word "calm."

    (c) Play Heavy Metal music turned up to high volume and think about something which makes me angry.

3. How do I prepare for a social event where others will be smoking?

    (a) Accept "just the one" cigarette to prove that I'm a non-smoker.

    (b) Drink more alcohol in order to make myself immune from the temptation to smoke.

    (c) Use self-hypnosis before the event and engage in mental rehearsal so that I see, hear and feel myself in my imagination enjoying the event and staying a non-smoker throughout.

4. If I face an unexpected difficulty in life, how do I get through that and remain a non-smoker?

    (a) Put myself into self-hypnosis and ask, "How do I successfully find a solution to this situation?" and let my unconscious mind come up with answers and ideas to move forward.

    (b) Ask myself, "Why can't I handle this kind of thing?"

(c)   Focus my attention on all the worst aspects of the difficulty.

5.   What is a useful way of managing stress at work?

(a)   Reflect on how out of control I feel.

(b)   Think of stress as a numerical scale from 100 to zero and use self-hypnosis to put myself into a state corresponding to the most useful number on that scale.

(c)   Spend my wages on gambling when off-duty in order to distract my mind.

6.   If I face a "moment of temptation" in which a smoker offers me a cigarette while socialising, what is a useful way of getting through that while remaining a non-smoker?

(a)   Decide to be only a "social smoker" and accept the cigarette.

(b)   Express hostility towards the smoker offering the cigarette.

(c)   Recognise that I only need to take a decision for the present moment, decide to choose the benefits of being a non-smoker, say, "No thanks, I don't smoke," and allow the conversation to move on.

7.   What is a good habit to adopt with regard to alcohol in order to stay a non-smoker?

(a)   Learn to appreciate quality alcoholic drinks, focus attention on, and enjoy, each sip, so that I get more pleasure out of less alcohol.

(b)   Give up alcohol completely.

(c)   Increase my consumption of the cheapest and nastiest alcoholic drinks.

8.   What is the best way to stay slim now that I am a non-smoker?

(a)   Eat only processed foods with high artificial sugar content.

(b)   Respond only to "mouth hunger" by eating whenever I salivate.

(c)   Eat only in response to stomach hunger, eat mainly water-rich foods which are close to nature, eat slowly like a gourmet, paying attention to and enjoying the food, and stop eating when my stomach gives the signal that it is full up.

9. How do I deal with any cravings that might occur in the two weeks after I stop smoking?

    (a) Recognise that any cravings only last for ten seconds, and will anyway become fewer and weaker until they disappear after two weeks, and distract my mind for those ten seconds by an action such as eating an apple or drinking water.

    (b) Express anger towards those around me.

    (c) Eat sweets, chocolate and cream cakes in order to distract my attention from the cravings.

10. How can I usefully deal with the higher level of energy that I now have as a non-smoker?

    (a) Lie awake sleepless all night.

    (b) Play computer games.

    (c) Take up some form of regular light exercise, such as walking rather than driving or using public transport.

                                            Score: [number] out of 10.

Note that with question 7, both (a) and (b) are correct answers. (Presumably it is unnecessary to give the answers for the other questions.) After the seminar, mark these questionnaires and add them to the file that you keep on each training session.

It is also recommended that you write a trainer's log of each event, describing how the attendees responded to each stage of the seminar and mentioning anything noteworthy that happened. Keep this log permanently. If the company management asks to see it, you will be able to send them a copy. It will also be useful to you as you continuously develop and improve your seminars. If a participant asks an unusual question which you do not know the answer to, seek out the answer after the event by consulting the Internet, books or people with the relevant knowledge. That way, if someone at a future seminar asks a similar question, you can immediately give the answer.

3. Behaviour

This is what management will be most interested in! If the training is successful, the attendees will stop smoking during it and stay stopped permanently, using the techniques you have taught them to deal with every conceivable situation. In case of any relapses, it is essential to offer backup, such as attendance at another seminar or a one-to-one session, for attendees who request it, whether or not they have relapsed. Both you and the company's management will want to keep accurate records of how the seminar has affected behaviour. It is advisable, by arrangement with the management, to check back after a reasonable length of time, such as a month or three months, to ensure that everyone who attended your seminar either stopped smoking successfully or has had the opportunity to make use of back-up support.

By keeping accurate records, you will know how effective your seminar is. With the permission of the company's management, you can also use the data to write up a case study which you can present as evidence to new potential corporate clients who may want to see proof of the effectiveness of your programme.

4. Results

5. Return on investment

6. Intangible benefits

For each of these levels of evaluation, the management is likely to do the evaluation for themselves with little involvement from the trainer. You might ask them for a written statement as to the results they have obtained as a result of your programme, and, if they are willing to provide it, for permission to quote the statement in your communications with other potential corporate clients as part of a case study.

Keeping documents

The management will want copies of the documents relating to the training in order to put them in the personnel files which they hold on each employee. It is essential to provide the management with these records, as employees have the legal right under the Data Protection Act 1998 to see all files their present or former employers have on them. The management is also likely to require the documents relating to your training in order to monitor the overall level of training activity, to assess the effectiveness of training, build a record of an employee's learning and achievements, and to build a database of what external trainers have done. Those documents may also be needed to meet the requirements of the company's insurers or health care providers, a quality programme such as IiP, or statutory bodies such as the Health and Safety Executive.

With the permission of each company's management, you should also keep copies of the documents relating to your training yourself. As you build your corporate smoking cessation service in the medium to long term, they will be a useful record of how that service continuously develops. Also, it is possible that a document may be needed at some point in the future for insurance or legal purposes. If you are short of storage space and find the papers piling up, then use the services of a digital storage company who will scan all the documents onto CD-Roms which take up minimal storage space. If your files contain the names of the employees who have attended your seminars, the law may require you to register under the Data Protection Act. Visit the website of the Information Commissioner at www.informationcommissioner.gov.uk to find out more.

Even when you are regularly delivering your seminars to the corporate world, you should continue to seek to improve and refine them. As well as tailoring them to the particular company and its employees, you can always add new therapeutic techniques which you learn from books, seminars and DVDs, and test them for effectiveness. By continually innovating, refining and reviewing your group seminar, it will become ever more effective, and remain fresh and dynamic both for you and for the attendees.

Chapter 15

A parting message: Life's journey

There are further opportunities to add value to the lives of your clients. It is often difficult to time a hypnotherapy session exactly, whether with an individual client or with a group. Often you will find that you finish five, ten or fifteen minutes before the end of the appointed time. Rather than simply finish early, it is recommended to use this time to give the maximum possible added value to the individual or group with whom you are working. What follows is an induction designed especially for use whenever you have a few minutes to spare at the close of the session. It draws on the subject's previous experiences of success in life, and aims to establish mental and physical harmony and provide a metaphor for the future course of life.

Life's journey

"And this is where your journey really begins …

"So now that it's all over, and you have achieved what you set out to achieve when you came here today, you can just take it easy for a moment. Can you remember those other moments in your life just after you achieved something really monumental. Was there a particular set of exams or tests that you passed, perhaps something to do with studying or with your career? And how did you feel the moment after you learned that you'd passed those tests? Was there a particular offer of a place at some college or school, or when you got a job you really wanted, or sold something to a really important customer? And what about when you got your first swimming certificate – your cycling proficiency test – your driving test? And perhaps there have been other great moments in life when you've felt just like that. And maybe you can imagine watching those scenes of yourself on a TV screen, just like home videos which have been edited together, observing the expression on your face in those moments of triumph and pride, noticing the way you hold your body, the sound of your voice. Success, triumph, achievement, from being a young child, through being a teenager, entering the adult world. And as you watch those scenes on that home video, just let yourself step inside your own body inside that screen any time you like and feel the way you feel in that moment, see what you can see with your own eyes and hear what you can hear with your own ears, and really notice the difference. And can you experience that more vividly with your eyes open or closed? That's right.

"You can be very pleased about the wonderful transformation which you have achieved. You can be pleased that your body, your unconscious mind, is also pleased. Did you know that each organ of your body has its own identity? It's a very interesting thing. They found that when a kidney transplant takes place, the person who has received that transplant can, in their dreams, learn a lot about the life of the person who donated the kidney. The kind of person they were, their age, their experiences, their thoughts. It's as if every part of the human body somehow has an identity, and in this very relaxed state, now you've done your body this wonderful favour, it's time to explore your body, time to welcome this wonderful transformation to health in this very relaxed state.

"When you were a child, you learned to use your imagination, and that power of imagination is still there inside. There was once a science fiction film called *Fantastic Voyage* – I don't know if you ever saw it. And what they did was that they got a little vehicle, something like a spaceship or a diving bell with people on board. They shrank it down to a tiny, microscopic size. Then they put it inside a living human body, and in that kind of spaceship they could explore the whole of that body. I wonder if you can imagine doing that now. Imagine yourself in a kind of spaceship being shrunk down to a tiny microscopic size.

"In a moment I will count down in a series of fractions, from one-half down to one-thousandth. And with each fraction, I'd like you to imagine that you are shrinking down to that fraction of your original size. Something like Alice in the story, in which she shrinks down so that she can get through that little doorway. And with each fraction, your body will become more and more relaxed, your mind wandering, so that by the time you are one thousandth of your original size, you'll be in that same relaxed, tranquil, peaceful, creative state of inner awareness that you've already entered several times today. So ready: one-half – shrinking down to half your full size, those muscles loosening and unwinding. One quarter – reducing to a quarter your original size, as your body relaxes deeper and deeper. One tenth – tinier and tinier, while your breathing slows, and all the areas of tension in your body melt away as those muscles relax more and more. One hundredth – deeper and deeper relaxed, everything slowing down in a pleasant, healthy way. One thousandth, and now so deeply relaxed, and so tiny that you could move through the human body without even being noticed.

"Can you imagine now exploring your own body, encased in that little spaceship that keeps you completely safe and protected. Going deep inside, maybe going through the mouth, that vast cavern with that huge tongue underneath, being swallowed in a glass of water, going down the throat, deep down into the digestive system, surrounded by unfamiliar vast shapes, hearing the pounding of the human heart, being aware of the rhythm of the pulse. Inside this spaceship you can travel to every part of your body. And you can find those parts of your body which have benefited the most from the fact that you are now a healthy non-smoker. You can ask those organs of your body how they feel about this wonderful transformation.

"So first we'll go to the lungs. You can be aware of that vast, powerful rhythm of breathing of those lungs filled with air from the bottom to the top. You can explore those lungs. You can see how they're so clean and pink. Those lungs have got rid of those last vestiges of coal tar. You can ask your lungs now how they feel about that. Listen to what your lungs have to say and learn from that answer.

"Then you can travel to your heart. Be aware of that powerful beating, that rhythm pumping that blood through every part of your body. Your heart has now been freed from that burden. So it's so much easier for it to do its task of pumping, creating, sending that blood out to every part of your body. Ask your heart now how it feels about this wonderful transformation and listen to your heart's answer.

"And you can go to your throat now. Be aware of that constant flow of air flowing through that mighty throat. Ask your throat how it feels about the fact that it's so much easier to breathe. Listen to your throat's answer.

"And you can explore now throughout the whole of your body, exploring your bloodstream, flowing down a vein, an artery. Notice the quality of your blood, how it's rich and red now there's so much more oxygen flowing through that red blood. Wonderful oxygen, bringing life and nutrients to every part of your body. Ask your bloodstream how it feels now this wonderful transformation towards health has been achieved, and listen to your bloodstream's answer.

"And you can explore through other parts of your body too. See them, feel them, hear them, ask them about their experience of this wonderful improvement. You'll find that your body works in harmony now and that you can repeat this wonderful tour of your body any time you like.

"Your body is the vessel that carries you through life. So see the vessel of your body, setting out to sea, leaving the shore, making sure that it's seaworthy. And when your vessel, perhaps a liner, or other kind of ocean-going boat, or maybe a yacht with both sails and a powerful engine, needs attention, because it's a bit dilapidated, the engine rusting, paint peeling, leaks in the hull, generally looking downbeat and weather-beaten, dirt in the engine, then it's time to do some work. If you wanted to take a boat across the ocean, you'd want to restore that boat. You'd want to fix those leaks, plug them up solidly, take out the engine, recondition that engine, throw away the rusted parts and put in new clean parts, chuck out all that dirt, put in some new equipment. You'd want to paint the sides, spruce it up, give it a new interior, patch up the sails, until finally that boat's good and seaworthy, the crew is ready to take you out on the ocean. And you can look forward to a wonderful cruise across that ocean. You'd take that boat from the dry dock to the harbour. You'd make sure you have all the supplies you need.

"Take that boat out on a calm sea, really enjoy that freedom of movement, the ocean waves bobbing that boat up and down, that vast stretch of expanse of blue, stretching to the horizon, the blue cloudless sky, a calm day at sea as that powerful reconditioned engine moves that boat quickly forward through the water leaving a long trail of white froth on the sea behind, going out into the ocean as the sun sinks, the vast night sky comes out and a high wind blows, those waves get bigger and stronger, buffeting that boat. A choppy sea. It's good to see that boat is seaworthy – it can survive that choppiness even if a huge storm breaks, rain cascades down, you can be tossed up and down but whatever the sea does, you know that that boat will remain afloat, remain upright. You know that that boat is seaworthy because you have prepared it.

"You have all the supplies you need to ride through choppy seas, stormy seas, until finally the sun comes up, the storm breaks, the seas become calm, so that once again you're moving forward in that wonderful reconditioned boat, confident and happy that you can keep going for as long as you like. So that you can find yourself enjoying every aspect of your life more and more, learning to trust your inner abilities, achieving things which maybe you thought could never be achieved, finding yourself relating to other people in a more relaxed, authentic way, gaining fulfilment out of simple pleasures in life. Living your own life.

"And during all this talking, since you first heard the sound of my voice, your unconscious mind has been learning and responding in a way which is unique and authentic and proper for you. So to tie everything together, I'd like to ask the unconscious mind now to take just a few silent moments to interpret, to learn, in a way which is truly proper and authentic for you. So just take a few moments to do that, starting now. (Remain silent for whatever length of time is warranted.)

"And this wonderful process of learning, understanding and transformation can continue today, tonight and in the days ahead. And in a few moments I'm going to invite you to return to the here and now. You'll hear me count up from one thousandth to full size. You'll grow back up to each size with each fraction, until when I say, 'full size', your eyes will open and you'll be fully wide awake. You'll wake up feeling refreshed, happy, confident, with a strong sense of achievement, looking forward to the future and with your eyes open when I say, 'full size'. So ready – one thousandth – one hundredth – growing and expanding with every moment – one tenth – getting bigger and bigger – one quarter – about the size of one of the little people – one-half – larger and larger – full size. Wide awake – wide awake."

Appendix 1

Workplace smoking and the law

In the United States, the question of smoking is determined at the state or municipal level, not by the federal government; therefore, smoking policies are instituted on a state-by-state basis.

In the United Kingdom, increasingly, legislation has sought to influence companies into taking a greater degree of responsibility for the health of their staff. The Health and Safety at Work Act 1974 established that employers have a duty of care to their workforce, and requires them to provide instruction to ensure the health and safety at work of all employees. More recently, the Health Act 2006, which came into force in England, Wales and Northern Ireland in 2007, prohibits smoking in virtually all enclosed workplaces. A similar law was introduced in Scotland in 2006.

Under the Health Act 2006, every time a Health and Safety Executive inspector catches an employee smoking in the workplace, or finds evidence that smoking has taken place, such as discarded cigarette butts, the company will receive a stiff fine, even if the management did not know about the smoking and had previously instructed staff to obey the law.

This Act poses a challenge for many companies which had hitherto provided smoking rooms for the use of smoking staff during their breaks. Companies in the leisure, entertainment, hotel and catering sectors, where smoking by staff and customers in workplaces was widespread before the Act, will have to adapt their corporate culture significantly and quickly in order to comply with the new laws.

In April 2007, the National Institute for Health and Clinical Excellence (NICE) launched Public Health Intervention 5, which includes advice on the support that companies should give to those employees who want to quit smoking. NICE points out that smoking is the largest preventable cause of death in the United Kingdom, costs the National Health Service £1.5 billion annually, and costs industry an estimated £5 billion in lost productivity, fire damage and absenteeism as a result of smoking-related illnesses such as cardiovascular disease and respiratory diseases. According to NICE, the average smoking employee is off sick thirty-three hours more per year than a non-smoking colleague. The NICE guidance recommends that employers provide smoking cessation support in the workplace, both in order to help those employees who want to become non-smokers, and also to help both employers and employees stay on the right side of the new laws. The guidance points out that a healthier, non-smoking workforce means increased productivity, so that employers and staff alike benefit.

In launching the initiative, Catherine Law, chair of the Public Health Interventions Advisory Committee (PHIAC) at NICE, said:

> "Smoking is a public health priority as well as the principal cause of inequalities in life expectancy between rich and poor in this country. The new legislation on smoke free workplaces will prevent exposure to second-hand smoke in the workplace but it also provides the opportunity to create an environment which makes it easier to quit for those who want to. Providing support at work will reach people who may not usually seek help to stop smoking, such as young men."

Dr David Sloan, PHIAC member at NICE, a public health specialist and former general practitioner, said:

> "We know that overall around three out of four smokers want to quit. It's important for employees and their representatives to work with employers on what support they need to give up smoking, and to encourage their employers to make that support available. Along with the health benefits of stopping smoking, employees who quit will give themselves an instant 'pay rise' – a 20-a-day smoker will save nearly £2,000 a year by stopping smoking."

Mary Broughton, health and safety chair of the Federation of Small Businesses (FSB), said:

> "Small businesses recognise the need to support their staff in the workplace. Given the forthcoming ban on smoking in enclosed workplaces this support can now extend to helping employees who wish to stop smoking. This situation works out well for employers and employees. It will improve the health of staff and the productivity of businesses. It will also ensure that the new smoking laws are not broken. This advice from NICE has come at just the right time and we at the FSB are pleased to recommend it to our members."[1]

Appendix 2

Benefits of smoking cessation seminars to organisations

In promoting smoking cessation seminars to corporate decision-makers, it is essential to educate them as to the benefits – for the company as well as individual employees – of achieving a smoke-free workforce. These benefits are both tangible – and financially measurable – and intangible. The first task of a provider of corporate smoking cessation seminars is to demonstrate how the corporate client will benefit in both areas by making use of such services. It is also necessary to build credibility by proving that the hypnotherapy approach is successful in achieving the results desired.

Tangible benefits of a non-smoking workforce to a company

Those employees who smoke cost the average employer £1,800 each every year in lost productivity. On average, smokers are absent through sickness 32 percent more than their non-smoking colleagues. Time and motion studies have found that smoking breaks taken by smokers above and beyond the official breaks granted to all employees add up to an average of thirty minutes a day, or no less than eighteen days per smoker per year. These costs are recovered over time once those employees become non-smokers and improve their performance.

Smokers face early retirement at a far higher rate than non-smokers, due to the damage they have done to their health. Death rates before retirement are also significantly higher for smokers than non-smokers. This means that companies lose skills, knowledge and corporate continuity by the sickness or death of some of their most experienced staff. Providing the opportunity for those employees to become non-smokers can reduce much of those costs.

In addition, employers have to pay higher insurance premiums for every employee who smokes. The insurance companies know the risks all too well. The larger the proportion of the workforce which becomes non-smokers, the lower the insurance costs.

Intangible benefits of a smoke-free workforce

A company which provides the opportunity for its employees to become non-smokers gains significant benefits which are intangible, but nevertheless real. A company's actions on smoking are likely to be in harmony with its organisational objectives. Most companies have written objectives, many of which include a commitment to the personal and professional development of employees.

A non-smoking workforce also means greater job satisfaction. Most smokers know how much better off they will be, at work and off-duty, once they become non-smokers. Healthy workers with a strong sense of individual well-being enjoy higher morale and contribute to the general quality of the workplace environment. An enhanced team spirit is created when everyone in the workplace becomes a non-smoker. Employees appreciate the company's support in enabling them to quit smoking, and feel a greater sense of mutual support and company loyalty. People spend a lot of time at work, tend to define themselves largely by their jobs, and are influenced by the group environment of the workplace. They are more likely to be influenced by the positive encouragement to become non-smokers by their managers and co-workers. The fact that all workplaces are now smoke-free by law adds to that supportive environment.

In an increasingly competitive business world, corporate image becomes all the more vital as an intangible. A circle of smokers outside the front entrance creates a poor first impression to customers arriving at a company's premises, particularly if the breeze blows a cloud of smoke in their faces as they reach the door. Those smokers can create noise, litter and a nuisance for neighbouring companies and residences as well. A non-smoking workforce therefore enhances the company's image.

Increasingly, companies are becoming aware of the importance of corporate social responsibility. Providing the opportunity for the enhancement of health and well-being among employees is an example. Companies that commit to their employees' health present a responsible image within the workplace and in the wider community. This in turn helps to attract and maintain the best employees. A business which is seen to be proactive in supporting its workforce becomes a business where people want to work.

Appendix 3

The use of music for relaxation

Mankind has always used music as a means of achieving altered states of consciousness and group identity. In developing his system of accelerated learning, Georgi Lozanov found that playing Baroque music composed between 1700 and 1750 (the "purest" Baroque music) caused greater alpha wave activity in the brain, greater left and right brain coordination and much improved learning and recall. Each of my individual clients receives a copy of the CD "Baroque music for self-hypnosis", which I produced, with a recommendation to listen to it while doing self-hypnosis. The CD consists of orchestral pieces by C. P. E. Bach, Händel and Vivaldi, performed by the Hypnotic Orchestra, conducted by Steven Fox, and organ music by Buxtehude, J. S. Bach, Tunder, Krebs and Böhm. The pieces were selected partly because of their relaxing and hypnotic effect, and partly because they are not too familiar to the public. This music forms the backing for the hypnotic inductions on my own series of self-hypnosis CD sets.

Be wary of giving clients Baroque pieces that are too familiar, as they may be anchors to disempowering states. For instance, Vivaldi's *Four Seasons* is commonly used when people are put "on hold" on the telephone – an anchor most definitely to be avoided.

The definitive Baroque solo keyboard piece is J. S. Bach's *Goldberg Variations*. There is a story that Bach was commissioned to compose this piece by an aristocrat who had trouble sleeping. Many creative individuals listen to it every day. My favourite version available on CD is the relatively spirited performance by the pianist Ekaterina Dershavina.

For the introductory music at group or corporate events, I play relaxing music which is likely to suit the tastes of most attendees. This would be "Baroque music for self-hypnosis" for those who are likely to enjoy classical music. For those who are more likely to prefer contemporary music, the theme tune for the film *Somewhere in Time*, composed by John Barry shortly after the deaths of his parents, has a remarkably dissociative affect. A group who are spiritually inclined might be suited to the vocals of the Ecumenical Community at Taizé, a Gregorian chant or Indonesian (Balinese or Javanese) trance music. Ambient music, which is designed to be either listened to consciously or to be played in the background without conscious attention, is also suitable for introductory music.

Other choices are ambient music, such as that by Brian Eno, Vangelis and Mike Oldfield. However, avoid playing Oldfield's *Tubular Bells*, which was later used as the theme tune to the film *The Exorcist* – not exactly an anchor for the states we want to induce.

Later in the group session, when the main hypnotic trance is induced, I play music specifically created to induce trance. My previous choice was Ormond McGill and Tom Silver's *Hypno-Music*, but more recently I have preferred Dick and Tara Sutphen's *Astral Journey*, which is designed to bring the listener from beta, through alpha, to theta state.

List of CDs

Title	Artist	Composer	Label	Catalogue no.	Availability
Astral Journey	Dick and Tara Sutphen	Dick and Tara Sutphen	Red Ball on Blue Water	RB302	New Age shops or www.dicksutphen.com
Goldberg Variations	Ekaterina Dershavina	J. S. Bach	Arte Nova Classics	7-321 34011 2	Music stores
Somewhere in Time	John Barry	John Barry (with one track by Sergei Rachmaninov)	BGO/MCA	BGOCD222	Music stores
Laudate Omnes Gentes	Ecumenical Community of Taizé	Jacques Berthier and Taizé	Auvidis	T-566	Music stores
Ommadawn	Mike Oldfield	Mike Oldfield	Virgin	7-43 8 49370 2 7	Music stores
Islands	Mike Oldfield	Mike Oldfield (Track 1 – "Wind Chimes" – is based on Balinese trance music).	Virgin	7-43 8 49383 2 1	Music stores
The Songs of Distant Earth	Mike Oldfield	Mike Oldfield	WEA	4509 98542 2	Music stores
Hypno-Music	Ormond McGill and Tom Silver	Ormond McGill and Tom Silver	Silver Institute	15097	www.anglo-american.co.uk
Baroque music for self-hypnosis	Hypnotic Orchestra, Daniel Cook, David Pipe	Various	CMS	CE11	www.selfhypnosiscd.co.uk
Stop Smoking Today	David Botsford	Various	CMS	CE1	www.selfhypnosiscd.co.uk
Ambient 1: Music for Airports (the original ambient music album)	Brian Eno	Brian Eno	Virgin	7-43 8 66495 2 2	Music stores
The Best of Vangelis	Vangelis	Vangelis (Track 1 – 'Spiral' is particularly useful. Track 11 – "Dervish D" is based on the mystical trance music of the whirling dervishes of Sufism)	BMG	7-321 939772	Music stores

Anglo-American Books also offer CDs by numerous artists suitable for these purposes.

Appendix 4

Suggestions for further reading

Here is a list of my favourite books about smoking cessation, hypnosis and related techniques. It is not intended to be a complete bibliography on the subjects discussed in the present volume. There are plenty of worthwhile books on these subjects which are not mentioned here.

Hypnosis

All works by Milton H. Erickson. Although Erickson wrote many thousands of pages, he intentionally never wrote a book specifically on "Ericksonian hypnotherapy" because he wanted his students to develop their own individual styles. The four-volume collection of *The Seminars, Workshops and Lectures of Milton H. Erickson*, edited by Ernest L. Rossi, et al, (first published 1983), Free Association Books, London, 1998, contains transcripts of his live events; its spontaneous oral style is readable and accessible. The four-volume *Collected Papers of Milton H. Erickson on Hypnosis*, edited by Ernest L. Rossi, Irvington Publishers, New York, 1980, is an invaluable reference source, but much denser and not suitable to be read all the way through. Both are now available on one CD-Rom from the Anglo American Book Company Ltd.

There are numerous books describing Erickson's methods written by others. The classic summary of Erickson's approach to hypnosis is Richard Bandler and John Grinder, *Trance-formations*, Real People Press, Moab, Utah, 1981. It is currently out of print, and copies are difficult to locate and very expensive. A compact overview of Erickson's approach is William O'Hanlon and Michael Martin, *Solution-Oriented Hypnosis*, Norton, New York, 1992. A more substantial volume covering the same subject is Rubin Battino and Tom South, *Ericksonian Approaches*, Crown House Publishing, Bancyfelin, Carmarthen, 1999.

The classic work on authoritarian and direct hypnosis is Dave Elman, *Hypnotherapy* (originally titled *Findings in Hypnosis*, 1964), Westwood Publishing, Glendale, California, 1977. Elman's approach is particularly useful for groups.

The essential compilation of hypnotic techniques from a broad range of perspectives is D. Corydon Hammond (editor), *Handbook of Hypnotic Suggestions and Metaphors*, W. W. Norton/American Society of Clinical Hypnosis, New York, 1990.

NLP

Those aspects of NLP which are most useful to hypnotherapists derive from the early years, when the techniques were quick, simple and powerful. Two good introductions to NLP are Anthony Robbins, *Unlimited Power*, Simon and Schuster, New York, 1986, and Joseph O'Connor and John Seymour, *Introducing NLP*, first published 1990, Aquarian/HarperCollins, 1993. The most useful book for hypnotherapists written by the two founders of NLP is Richard Bandler and John Grinder, *Frogs into Princes*, Real People Press, Moab, Utah, 1979 (out of print).

Cognitive therapy

Out of the many books written by the two founders of cognitive therapy, two which explain the concepts succinctly but comprehensively are Aaron T. Beck, *Cognitive Therapy and the Emotional Disorders*, first published 1976, Penguin, London, 1989, and Albert Ellis and Catharine MacLaren, *Rational Emotive Behavior Therapy*, Impact Publishers, Atascadero, California, 1998.

Stress management

The definitive practical volume on stress management is Paul M. Lehrer and Robert L. Woolfolk (editors), *Principles and Practice of Stress Management*, 2nd edition, Guilford Press, New York, 1993, which contains chapters by the recognized leaders in the field. A more academic multi-author book is Alan Monat and Richard S. Lazarus (editors), *Stress and Coping*, 3rd edition, Columbia University Press, New York, 1991.

Yoga

Ormond McGill, *Hypnotism and Mysticism of India*, Westwood Publishing, Los Angeles, 1979 (originally titled *The Magic and Mysticism of India*, 1977), is a very well-informed first-hand account of yogic practices by the most accomplished lay hypnotist of the twentieth century. The same author's *Hypnotism and Meditation*, Westwood Publishing, Los Angeles, 1981, is a short work which fuses Western hypnosis with yoga to powerful effect. Both works are out of print and hard to find. Several yoga techniques are also included in the autobiography *The Amazing Life of Ormond McGill*, Crown House Publishing, 2003 (originally titled *Secrets of Dr Zomb*), which is in print, thanks to the excellent work of Crown House Publishing in keeping McGill's work available.

Books aimed at smokers who want to quit

The classic in this genre is Allen Carr, *The Easy Way to Stop Smoking*, Penguin, London, 1983. Neil Casey, *The Nicotine Trick*, Metro Publishing, London, 2002, also educates the smoker about the physical aspects in order to assist in quitting. Two books based on cognitive therapy are Gillian Riley, *How to Stop Smoking and Stay Stopped for Good*, Vermilion/Random House, 1992, and David F. Marks, *Overcoming Your Smoking Habit*, Constable and Robinson, London, 2005. A recent approach based on hypnosis and NLP is Paul McKenna, *Quit Smoking Today without Gaining Weight*, Bantam/Transworld/Random House, London, 2007.

Groups and corporate training

Virtually the only book exclusively devoted to group hypnotherapy is Hildegard Klippstein (editor), *Ericksonian Hypnotherapeutic Group Inductions*, translated by Twinky J. Steppacher-Ray, Brunner/Mazel, New York, 1991. It is a multi-author volume with many good ideas that can be adapted. A compact but thorough study of training in the corporate world is Steve Truelove, *Training in Practice*, first published 1997, Chartered Institute of Personnel and Development, London, 2006. Joseph O'Connor and John Seymour, *Training with NLP*, Thorsons/HarperCollins, London, 1994, shows how to use NLP to make training as effective as possible.

Endnotes

Introduction – The hypnotherapist and the smoking habit

(1)   Allen Carr, *Packing It in the Easy Way*, Michael Joseph/Penguin, London, 2004, pp. 74–75.

(2)   Ibid, pp. 110–111.

(3)   Ibid, pp. 112, 114.

(4)   Ibid, pp. 114–115

(5)   Ibid, p. 116.

(6)   Milton H. Erickson, "Deep hypnosis and its induction" (1952), in Ernest L. Rossi (editor), *The Collected Papers of Milton H. Erickson on Hypnosis*, vol. 1, Irvington Publishers, New York, 1980, p. 141.

(7)   Ibid, p.141.

(8)   Milton H. Erickson, "Utilizing unconscious processes in hypnosis" (1961), in Ernest L. Rossi, et al (editors), *The Seminars, Workshops and Lectures of Milton H. Erickson*, vol. 1, Free Association Books, London, 1998, p. 76.

Chapter 1 – The elements of transformation

No endnotes.

Chapter 2 – The nature and function of trance

(1)   Ernest L. Rossi, "Hypnosis and ultradian cycles", *American Journal of Clinical Hypnosis*, vol. 25, no. 1, July 1982, pp. 21–22.

(2)   Brian Inglis, *Trance*, Paladin/Grafton/Collins, London, 1989, p. 10.

(3)   Stephen Wolinsky with Margaret O. Ryan, *Trances People Live*, Bramble Company, Falls Village, Connecticut, 1991, pp. 6–7.

(4)   Milton H. Erickson, "Further experimental investigation of hypnosis" (1967), in Rossi (editor), *Collected Papers*, op cit, vol. 1, p. 42.

Chapter 3 – Fundamentals for success in smoking cessation

(1)   *New Scientist*, 31st October 1992, p. 3.

(2)   Neil Casey, *The Nicotine Trick*, Metro Publishing, London, 2002.

(3) Milton H. Erickson, "Therapeutic uses of altered orientation in hypnosis" (1962), in Rossi, et al (editors), *Seminars*, op cit, vol. 1, p. 116.

(4) Milton H. Erickson, "Hypnotic psychotherapy" (1948), in Rossi (editor), *Collected Papers*, op cit, vol. 4, pp. 35–48.

(5) Michael Yapko, "An interview with William S. Kroger, M.D.", recorded in 1987, *American Journal of Clinical Hypnosis*, vol. 38, no 3, January 1996, pp. 164–171.

(6) Chip and Dan Heath, *Made to Stick*, Random House, London, 2007, p. 211. In their book, Chip and Dan Heath refer to scientific research by Inna D. Rivkin and Shelley E. Taylor which supports this concept. They asked a group of UCLA students to think about a problem in their lives, and then asked one group, the event-simulators, to think through the chain of events that had led to the problem in detail. Another group, the outcome-simulators, had to imagine a positive outcome emerging from their problem, wondering what it would be like once the problem was behind them. Rivkin and Taylor conclude:

> "The event-simulation group – the people who simulated how the event unfolded – did better [at coping with their problems] on almost every dimension. Simulating past events is much more helpful than simulating future outcomes."

Chapter 4 – Preparing for the session

(1) A similar finding is described in Nalini Ambady and Robert Rosenthal, "Half a minute", *Journal of Personality and Social Psychology*, vol. 64, no 3, April 1993, pp. 431–441.

Chapter 5 – Starting the main smoking cessation session

(1) Edward Hall, *The Silent Language*, Doubleday, New York, 1959.

Chapter 6 – Educating the client to gain control

No endnotes.

Chapter 7 – The trance induction and after

(1) Paul Martin, *The Sickening Mind*, Flamingo/HarperCollins, London, 1998, p. 62.

(2) Erickson, "Hypnotic psychotherapy", op cit, pp. 35–48.

(3) Ernest Hilgard, foreword to David Waxman, *Hartland's Medical and Dental Hypnosis*, 1st published 1966, 3rd edition, Ballière Tyndall, London, 1989, p. *x*.

Chapters 8–11

No endnotes.

Chapter 12 – Building a one-to-one therapy practice

(1) Lady Liza Campbell, "Higher plane drifter", *Harpers and Queen*, November 2004, p. 136.

Chapter 13 – Running a group smoking cessation event

No endnotes.

Chapter 14 – Smoking cessation for the corporate market

(1) All quoted in Inglis, op cit, pp. 9–10.

(2) Quoted in Joseph O'Connor and John Seymour, *Training with NLP*, Thorsons/ HarperCollins, London, 1994, p. 103.

(3) For the Kirkpatrick model, see, for example: http://www.businessballs.com/ kirkpatricklearningevaluationmodel.htm

Chapter 15 – A parting message: Life's journey

No endnotes.

Appendix 1 – Workplace smoking and the law

(1) All quoted in National Institute for Health and Clinical Excellence, press release 2007/020 "Give quit smoking help at work, says NICE", 25th April 2007, www.nice.org.uk

Appendices 2–4

No endnotes.

Transcripts

(1) H. L. Mencken, *The American Language*, first published 1919, A. A. Knopf, New York, 4th edition, 1957, p. 573.

(2) Noam Chomsky, *Language and Problems of Knowledge*, MIT Press, Cambridge, Massachusetts, 1988, p. 36.

Index